U0290287

[英国]保罗·克莱纳曼 著 孙则书 译

牛津通识读本·

免疫系统

The Immune System

A Very Short Introduction

译林出版社

图书在版编目（CIP）数据

免疫系统／（英）保罗·克莱纳曼（Paul Klenerman）著；孙则书译.
--南京：译林出版社，2021.7（2023.7重印）
（牛津通识读本）
书名原文：The Immune System: A Very Short Introduction
ISBN 978-7-5447-8625-6

Ⅰ.①免…　Ⅱ.①保…　②孙…　Ⅲ.①医学－免疫学　Ⅳ.①R392

中国版本图书馆 CIP 数据核字（2021）第 061439 号

The Immune System: A Very Short Introduction, First Edition by Paul Klenerman
Copyright © Paul Klenerman, 2017
The Immune System: A Very Short Introduction, First Edition was originally published in
English in 2017. This licensed edition is published by arrangement with Oxford University
Press. Yilin Press, Ltd is solely responsible for this bilingual edition from the original work
and Oxford University Press shall have no liability for any errors, omissions or inaccuracies
or ambiguities in such bilingual edition or for any losses caused by reliance thereon.
Chinese and English edition copyright © 2021 by Yilin Press, Ltd
All rights reserved.

著作权合同登记号　图字：10-2020-86 号

免疫系统　　［英国］保罗·克莱纳曼／著　　孙则书／译

责任编辑　　陈　锐
装帧设计　　景秋萍
校　　对　　戴小娥
责任印制　　董　虎

原文出版　Oxford University Press, 2017
出版发行　译林出版社
地　　址　南京市湖南路 1 号 A 楼
邮　　箱　yilin@yilin.com
网　　址　www.yilin.com
市场热线　025-86633278
排　　版　南京展望文化发展有限公司
印　　刷　江苏扬中印刷有限公司
开　　本　890 毫米 × 1260 毫米　1/32
印　　张　8
插　　页　4
版　　次　2021 年 7 月第 1 版
印　　次　2023 年 7 月第 2 次印刷
书　　号　ISBN 978-7-5447-8625-6
定　　价　39.00 元

序 言

苏 冰

　　人们对免疫学的认识,源于人类千百年来对抗瘟疫流行的不懈努力。1796年,英国医生爱德华·詹纳发明了用于预防天花的牛痘疫苗,由此开创了现代免疫学的时代。免疫学作为一门年轻的学科,包含新的分析技术、新的工程实践,以及我们逐步对其本质的理解。高速发展的现代社会曾经乐观地估计,抗生素和疫苗能够让人类不再担忧感染性疾病,大量的医药领域研发资源被集中到了心血管疾病、神经退行性疾病以及癌症等人类慢性病当中。而2020年年初一场新型冠状病毒的大流行一下子让大家意识到,人类在不断演化、更新迭代的大自然面前仍然束手无策。因此,越来越多的有识之士意识到加强免疫学,尤其是感染免疫学研究发展的紧迫性和重要性。同时,免疫学界也意识到,免疫学的进一步发展,需要更多其他领域的专业人士来提供属于他们领域的见解,从而为免疫学的进一步发展提供宝贵思路和意见。因此,一份深入浅出的读本既可以帮助有志于将自己的技术背景投入免疫学研究的专业人士,亦可为希望了解免疫学大致进展的普罗大众打开一扇通往免疫学认知的窗。

　　牛津通识读本《免疫系统》正是这样一本科普读物，它致力于让试图获得基础免疫学知识的大专院校学生和普罗大众了解和认识免疫学，尤其是当代免疫学的最新发展方向。本书从最原始的免疫体系（同时也是最热门、最前沿的研究领域）细菌抗噬菌体的CRISPR系统开始，逐步介绍到无脊椎动物中的"模式识别受体"，以及脊椎动物的"适应性免疫系统"。这种以生物演化入手逐步展开介绍的方式，更有助于不甚了解免疫学的读者从生物学的视角深入理解认知免疫学。后续篇章则以免疫识别、免疫记忆、免疫耐受等免疫系统的基本功能为抓手，逐步展开讲解现代免疫学对基础原理与临床疾病发生发展的认知。本书的一大特点是，它除了对基础原理进行阐述之外，还融汇免疫学知识于疾病的阐释当中，从而进一步帮助读者理解免疫学，尤其是貌似枯燥的免疫学知识与自己切身经历的疾病之间的联系。此外，本书还进一步探讨了免疫学的前沿应用领域，如：新型疫苗、细胞治疗、单克隆抗体治疗、免疫系统年轻化等新方向，为希望进入这一领域的学者提供了可行的课题思路与研究方向。

　　本书的作者保罗·克莱纳曼，是牛津大学纳菲尔德医学院免疫学教授、威康信托基金会高级临床研究员、牛津大学生物医学研究中心的免疫课题主任。克莱纳曼教授长期从事感染性疾病，尤其是丙型肝炎病毒慢性感染和疫苗反应的相关研究工作，对肝脏CD161阳性黏膜相关恒定T细胞，尤其是这一细胞对宿主防御以及免疫病理当中的作用具有深入认知。他还从事对丙型肝炎病毒的免疫防御机制，尤其是腺病毒疫苗激活的T细胞

"记忆膨胀"的研究，对适应性免疫在宿主防御当中的作用有较为深入、细致的认知。他的生活与研究经历为此书的最终成功问世提供了充分保障。

免疫系统的稳态平衡是人体健康的核心环节，它的失调也直接造成了很多疾病的发生。除因新冠肺炎而引起全社会关注的感染免疫之外，现代免疫学的另一核心领域——肿瘤免疫的研究也正开展得方兴未艾，并已获得诺贝尔奖垂青。这表明免疫学在疫苗为人类攻克感染性疾病难关之后很可能会再下一城，为消灭万病之王做出自己的贡献。此外，也正如本书中所提到的，免疫学研究在帮助我们进一步理解衰老和炎症相关疾病方面也具有重要的潜在价值。

译林出版社从2008年就开始推出"牛津通识读本"丛书中文版，截至目前，已出版百余种，广泛涉及宗教、哲学、艺术、历史、法律、政治、商业、经济、数学、化学、天文、医学等领域。值此新型冠状病毒肺炎全球蔓延，疫苗接种全面铺开之时，这本《免疫系统》的推出无疑将有助于在民众当中普及现代免疫学知识，并为其他专业人士进入这一领域以进一步拓展免疫学的丰富内涵架设桥梁。

目　录

致　谢

　　我要感谢在此书写作过程中给我提供过帮助的所有人。首先，我要感谢牛津大学彼得·梅达沃楼转化胃肠病学组的同事尼克·普罗文、菲利帕·马修斯、苏西·杜纳奇和马特·比尔顿，他们阅读过本书的多版草稿。我要感谢克里斯·威尔伯格和阿尔巴·利伯雷为本书提供了生发中心的图片，感谢我的老同事菲利普·古尔德对我的包容并照料我的植物。我非常感谢来自牛津大学邓恩病理学学院的戴维·格里夫斯，他花了很多时间帮助和指导我，尤其是在巨噬细胞方面。我非常感谢我过去的免疫学老师：剑桥大学的赫尔曼·瓦尔德曼和艾伦·蒙罗，牛津大学的安德鲁·麦克迈克尔和罗德尼·菲利普斯，苏黎世大学的汉斯·亨加特纳和罗尔夫·辛克纳吉（以及他的病毒），是他们为我带来了这个课题，并以某种方式为本书中的观点做出了贡献。我必须感谢那些为我本人及实验室提供资金支持的人和机构，尤其要感谢威康信托基金会，他们从一开始就通过奖学金计划支持了我的工作。我还要感谢英国国家健康研究所

（资助了牛津大学生物医学研究中心）、牛津大学马丁学院、英国医学研究理事会、美国国立卫生研究院和英国癌症研究中心，它们对传染和免疫中的不同项目提供了大力支持。最后，我要感谢我的家人——我的妻子莎莉，我的孩子汤姆和艾玛——感谢他们带给我的所有爱、热情和活力，感谢他们让我有能力解释清楚本书的内容。我想把这本书献给我的父母莱斯利·克莱纳曼和内奥米·克莱纳曼（父亲是牛津通识读本《人体解剖学》的作者，母亲是写作此书的灵感之源），他们从一开始就鼓励我写作本书，但在本书完成之前过世了。他们的记忆（免疫学及其他方面）将一直延续。

i

ii

缩略语表

AID	活化诱导胞嘧啶脱氨酶
AIDS	获得性免疫缺陷综合征
BCG	卡介苗
bNABs	广谱中和抗体
CAR-T	嵌合抗原受体T细胞
CF	囊性纤维化
CMV	巨细胞病毒
CRISPR	规律成簇的间隔短回文重复序列
CRP	C反应蛋白
CVID	常见变异型免疫缺陷
DAMPs	损伤相关的分子模式
EBV	爱泼斯坦-巴尔病毒
HBV	乙型肝炎病毒
HCV	丙型肝炎病毒
HIV	人类免疫缺陷病毒
HLA	人类白细胞抗原

HMBPP	4-羟基-3-甲基-2-丁烯基焦磷酸盐
HPV	人乳头瘤病毒
IBD	炎症性肠道疾病
IDO	吲哚胺脱氧酶
ILCs	先天淋巴细胞
LCMV	淋巴细胞性脉络丛脑膜炎病毒
LPS	脂多糖
MAIT	黏膜相关恒定 T
MHC	主要组织相容性复合体
Mtb	结核分枝杆菌
MS	多发性硬化症
NET	中性粒细胞外陷阱
NK	自然杀伤
NOD2	核苷酸结合寡聚化结构域蛋白2
PAMPs	病原体相关分子模式
PD-1	程序性死亡受体1
RA	类风湿性关节炎
RAG	重组活化基因
RSV	呼吸道合胞病毒
siRNA	短干扰核糖核酸
SIVs	猴免疫缺陷病毒
TB	结核病
TCR	T细胞受体
TGFb	组织生长因子
TLR	Toll样受体
TNFα	肿瘤坏死因子α

什么是免疫系统?

免疫系统与免疫力

大多数人都熟知免疫力这一概念。免疫力的主要含义是面对传染病时保持健康,换种比喻方式可理解为免除一些令人不快的税款。"Immunity"一词源自拉丁语,意为"不常见的"或"有特权的"。这种含义可能是人们通过日常观察所得出的:普通人容易感染疾病,而特殊的人则会受到保护或免于感染。

尽管在流行病(多数人被感染、少数人免于感染的情况)的语境下,免疫这一概念非常容易理解,然而它隐藏了一个鲜有人知的特征。如今,我们已经认识到是免疫系统让我们一直保持健康。免疫系统的基本要素对保持健康十分有效,只有当免疫系统存在缺陷时,我们才容易感染特定类型的疾病。换句话说,在进化过程中,免疫系统已经受千锤百炼,因此可以非常有效地对付许多传染性生物体,即通过将这些传染性生物体从体内清除或挡在体外而让个体不会罹患任何重大疾病。

新型病原体（可引起疾病的微生物体），尤其是跨物种感染人体的病原体（例如，埃博拉病毒），会给免疫系统带来一系列新的挑战——但幸运的是，设计免疫系统的目的就是为了克服这种难以预见的威胁。不过，还有许多其他生物体仅在免疫结构或防御系统受损或发育不足时（例如，在新生儿中）引起疾病，或者通过特定基因的突变而引起疾病。此类感染（例如，由某些类型的细菌和酵母菌引起的感染）通常被称为**机会性感染**（即，它们仅在某些条件下致病）。一个著名的案例就是"泡泡男孩"戴维·维特尔：他的免疫系统非常脆弱，即使简单的身体接触也可能让他置身于严重感染的风险之中。正是此类案例——"自然条件下的实验"，或是可在实验室条件下进行研究的突变——让我们了解了免疫系统的正常功能，这就是所谓的"日常"宿主防御。如果脱离本书语境，用乔尼·米切尔的话来说就是："当你失去时才知道自己拥有过什么。"

免疫系统不仅抵御来自外部的威胁，而且也抵御内部的威胁。免疫系统可视为一种用于维持体内现状的系统，即所谓的**体内平衡**。因此，当一种外部生物入侵体内时，就会激活免疫系统来消除它。然而，当个体内部出现异常的组织变化并形成癌症时（正常调节的组织转变为增长和定位不受自然控制的异常组织），免疫系统也会发挥作用，这一点正为越来越多的人所认识。在某些（非常罕见的）情况下，癌症实际上可能是由某种微生物引起的，例如，病毒与宫颈癌（人类乳头瘤病毒或HPV）和某些淋巴癌（淋巴瘤，由爱泼斯坦-巴尔病毒引起）的形成有关。在这种情况下，免疫系统有可能对引起癌症的病毒做出反应。在许多其他情况下，免疫系统也有可能识别出癌组织内部的变化。本书稍后会对这一识别方式的诸多制衡机制进行讨论，而现代免疫学最令人兴奋的特征之一，就是可以利用免疫反应为癌症提供全新的有效治疗方法。

免疫系统的另一个重要特征，可由其所抵御的微生物体的特性得知。与宿主相比，细菌和病毒的基因组（生命体中遗传物质的总量）相对较小，例如，某些细小病毒只能编码两个完整的基因，而与此相比，人类能编码大约两万个完整的基因。病毒的基因组可以是RNA或DNA，它们可以携带相同类型的遗传信息，只不过会表现出不同的病毒生活方式。病毒会大规模地快速复制这些基因组（在病毒感染期间，每毫升血液中可能会复制出数百万个病毒），这就使突变和自然选择过程可以快速进行。在某些情况下，病毒使用的复制机制甚至会加剧这种情况，因为某些RNA病毒的聚合酶（一种通过复制基因组从而复制病毒的蛋白质）缺乏校对功能。如果人类以这样的错误率复制其庞大的基因组，那将是一种灾难，但对于病毒而言，如果复制的基因组有缺陷，则很容易进行替换。

栖息在宿主细胞中的病毒，会利用宿主自身的机制将宿主的某些真实基因组整合至自身的基因组中。例如，感染了世界上大部分人口的巨细胞病毒（CMV）就已经把几个免疫基因整合至自己的基因组中，并进行修改而为己所用。显然，这种适应的主要动机是为了逃避宿主免疫系统，尤其是病毒会使用这种方法从而在单个宿主或种群中长期存在。这样做的结果是，宿主与病原体之间**共同进化**的过程延长了——在单个宿主中，病原体可以快速完成适应，甚至有可能在几天之内适应个体的免疫反应，例如HIV。

根据我们如何理解免疫系统，也可以推导出一个重要的结论：如果说病毒已经适应了通过诸如阻断化学信号或阻断整个细胞通路的方式来躲避宿主的免疫反应，或者有效对抗宿主免疫反应的某个方面，那么也就在很大程度上说明了在正常的宿主防御策略中存在特定的分子或通路，同时也说明了其所具有的局限性。就像安全服务可以利用黑客来测试网络的防御性能一样，研究病毒可以让我们了解大量关于正常免疫系统的功能以及如何操纵免疫系统的知识。罗尔夫·辛克纳吉和彼得·多赫蒂的合作研究方向就是如何通过淋巴细胞识别病毒，并因此获得了1996年的诺贝尔奖，而辛克纳吉则将病毒描述为免疫学"最好的老师"。

不同生物体中的免疫系统

所有生物体都具有某种形式的免疫力，其免疫力的形式取决于它们所生活的自然环境和所面临的威胁。人类与其他哺乳动物之间具有许多相似的免疫学特征，这就是免疫学家可以把小鼠免疫系统用作合理模型的原因之一。不过，复杂的宿主防御系统所存在的时间要久远得多，可能已经存在约三千万年。

让人感到意外的是，细菌（通常被视为入侵者而非宿主）本身具有一种十分复杂的免疫形式来抵御感染，这一点十分有趣。细菌会受到被称为**噬菌体**的特殊病毒的侵袭，噬菌体可以在细菌的DNA上"搭便车"。细菌则学会了通过CRISPR（规律成簇的间隔短回文重复序列）系统来保护自己。

CRISPR系统的工作机制是基于Cas分子家族（如Cas9）

的活性,这类分子可以使DNA断裂或产生"切口",从而阻断该DNA序列并有效清除基因。这些切口分子需要被引导从而实现上述效果,否则它们会破坏重要的宿主基因。不过,这些分子可以通过由CRISPR DNA序列生成的一组特定的核酸向导来实现上述机制,而这一核酸向导可以靶向针对入侵位点。这就使细菌能够有效地监管自身的DNA序列并对入侵基因做出反应。

细菌会故意在CRISPR区域捕获外源DNA序列,来靶向针对特定的噬菌体,从而适应其免疫系统(见图1),这就是CRISPR系统变得复杂的原因。尽管免疫反应中的识别策略各不相同,涉及的细胞多种多样,但生物体中的感染**识别**、宿主修饰、**特异性反应**及**长期记忆**等一系列步骤已经反映在人体的免疫系统中。

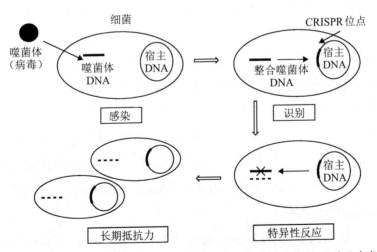

图1　细菌可以通过CRISPR/Cas系统对病毒产生特异性反应,该系统会复制出一个经过修饰的病毒序列(如虚线所示),细胞可以利用该序列来破坏入侵的噬菌体

5

虽然CRISPR/Cas系统作为细菌的宿主防御机制这一说法听起来十分有趣，但是我们也可以为己所用，将该系统应用于分子生物学。通过将CRISPR系统引入哺乳动物细胞，并利用针对目的基因设计的CRISPR向导对该系统进行指导，就可以非常有效地破坏或修复基因组。CRISPR/Cas系统刚被发现不久，但是它已经对基因组编辑领域产生了巨大的影响，具有巨大的科研前景及治疗潜力：最终，我们也许可以编辑人类的基因组。不过有趣的是，病毒可能已经先行一步——**拟菌病毒**是一种含有复杂基因组的巨型病毒，人们发现在拟菌病毒中已经出现类似CRISPR系统的迹象，用以保护其免受噬病毒体的侵害。

与动物、细菌一样，植物也容易受到病毒感染，它们也拥有自己的防御系统。植物中的RNA病毒可以通过被称为**RNA干扰**的过程进行降解：通过利用siRNA（短干扰RNA，一种RNA向导）和RISC（一种降解复合物），可以像CRISPR/Cas系统一样，对入侵的RNA进行靶向降解，而不影响宿主自身的RNA。这种RNA向导由植物产生并与入侵的病毒进行特异性结合，从而抑制病毒的复制。同样的，细胞生物学家可以利用这一生物学原理敲除特定宿主来源的基因，换句话说，就是抑制特定基因的蛋白质生成过程。与CRISPR/Cas系统一样，这里提到的RNA降解过程也具有治疗潜力；人们已经对人体内的基因敲除进行了各种尝试，比如抑制肝炎病毒和癌细胞的复制，甚至用于降低胆固醇水平。

这些例子表明，宿主防御可以在单个细胞内发生，从而保护宿主细胞的基因组。尽管人类自身的免疫系统不具有上述机制，但是这些机制对人类生物学有着重要意义。

其他具有悠久进化历史的机制，已经成为人类免疫力的重要组成部分。例如，Toll受体最初是由纽斯莱因-沃尔哈德和维斯豪斯在果蝇体内发现的（Toll在德语中是"惊讶"的意思，显然这表达了对此发现的惊叹）。Toll受体在昆虫的胚胎发育中起着重要作用，后来人们还发现Toll受体可以通过释放抗微生物蛋白和激活免疫细胞来启动防御真菌的免疫反应。人类拥有一系列类似的相关蛋白，被称为"Toll样受体"，可以发出信号并激活免疫反应。尽管就激活的细胞的多样性而言，其下游的影响在人体中更为复杂，但一开始的过程与果蝇中的起始过程非常相似（这一点将在第二章中做进一步讨论）。

这种模式化识别以及对于抗微生物防御机制的诱导，在许多生物体中都很常见，但是直到生物进化的后期（CRISPR/Cas系统是个例外），才开始出现具有经典适应性特征的免疫反应，即针对个体病原体产生的高度多样化反应。与人类免疫系统最为相似的首个免疫系统的例子就是无颌鱼类（例如，七鳃鳗）。这些动物具有生成病原体特异性受体的一种机制，这种受体与人体所用的受体有些相似，但又有所不同（请参见第三章）。有趣的是，无颌鱼类还会产生这些受体的可溶形式（相当于人体内的抗体）以及与细胞结合的形式（相当于人体内的T淋巴细胞）。从有颌鱼类开始，我们就可以看到一个明显的免疫系统的进化。

人体免疫系统

免疫系统不只是一组具有不同功能的特异性细胞，而是存在于人体的每个细胞中。因此，在提到人体免疫系统时，要注意不要忽视组织的作用,尽管免疫学家通常认为组织不具备"免疫学"上的意义(见图2)。例如,在宿主抵御细菌和病毒方面,皮肤起着特殊的作用。病毒需要利用活细胞进行复制,因此皮肤外表面上由死细胞层构成的"死亡之墙"阻止了许多感染的发生。只有少数病毒能够感染皮肤中的细胞,不过感染的也是位于皮肤深层的细胞:例如,人类乳头瘤病毒会引发良性疣从而导致宫颈癌等癌症。此外,皮肤还会通过分泌抗菌脂肪酸来抵御细菌。皮肤的破损则容易并发局部的细菌感染,对烧伤患者而言尤其如此。

尽管宿主竭尽全力创造一个毫无吸引力的体表环境,然而皮肤表面的实际情况却是多种微生物体相对和平地共处。在这

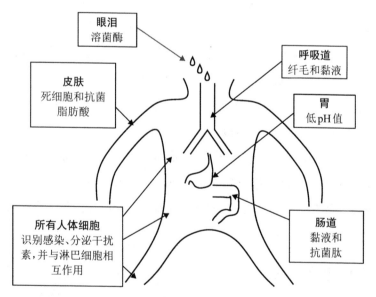

图2　所有人体细胞通过识别感染来增强人体的免疫力。此外,免疫系统还包括在体内外交界处形成关键屏障的离散结构以及明显属于免疫系统的其他结构

些微生物体中,有些会在其他部位引起严重的疾病。例如,**金黄色葡萄球菌**是一种令人恐惧的侵入性细菌,会对人体的许多器官造成严重的组织损伤,但是大约有四分之一的人类都在鼻孔处携带有这种细菌,却没有造成任何伤害。其他种类的葡萄球菌(例如,**表皮葡萄球菌**或凝固酶阴性葡萄球菌)所含有的侵袭性基因危害性较小,并自人类个体诞生起就寄生在人体的皮肤上。然而,即便是这些"共生体",当皮肤屏障被破坏时,它们也会进入人体的其他部位从而对人体造成严重的感染。例如,让这些细菌可以在皮肤上寄生的附着力,也可以让它们对塑料人工关节和心脏瓣膜造成长期感染。眼睛拥有专门的防御系统来保护角膜,眼泪中含有溶菌酶(这是由亚历山大·弗莱明发现的最早的抗菌分子之一,弗莱明后来还发现了青霉素),溶菌酶可以结合并破坏许多细菌。

皮肤是抵御潜在病原体的巨大的外部屏障,而这种外部的免疫屏障也存在于人体内部。上呼吸道和肺部是感染的多发部位,阅读本书的诸君将会了解鼻病毒感染是如何引起普通感冒的。皮肤可以形成具有清晰物理保护特性的多层屏障,但是与皮肤不同,上呼吸道和肺部仅仅受到薄薄的一层**黏膜**保护。肺部尤其如此,为了进行气体交换,它的内衬细胞(或上皮细胞)非常薄。呼吸道的免疫特征之一是一种物理性结构——纤毛"梯子",它的上皮细胞具有细小的毛状结构(纤毛),这些纤毛有节律地运动,从而使黏液沿着气道向上持续运动并排出肺部。因此,诸如细菌之类的侵入生物体被困在黏液中,并不断从敏感部位排出至上呼吸道中,而在上呼吸道中它们的危害性相对较小。

和皮肤一样，在通常情况下，上呼吸道的内容物并不是无菌的。人体的喉咙部位潜藏着许多危险的病毒，比如肺炎球菌，而肺炎球菌入侵肺组织就是引起肺炎的主要原因。在其功能因基因受损的罕见病（纤毛综合征）中，我们就可以看到纤毛"梯子"的重要性。缺少纤毛防御机制会导致由细菌引起的慢性肺部疾病（导致**支气管扩张**，破坏肺组织）。另一种影响黏膜-纤毛"梯子"的基因疾病是囊性纤维化（CF）。在这种疾病中，形成黏液的细胞泵存在缺陷，导致黏液变得过于黏稠。因此，具有CF基因缺陷的个体会反复发生肺部细菌感染。

黏膜防御一直延续到膈的下面，那里如果有事发生，宿主所面临的风险会更大。肠道含有数以万亿计的细菌——实际上，人体内90%的细胞都含有细菌。这种复杂的菌群或**微生物群**被肠道中薄薄的上皮细胞及其黏液层所阻隔。如果这些细菌穿过这层薄膜，就可能导致严重的疾病，如果出现肠穿孔则情况更为严重。一方面需要将免疫反应限制在肠道的正常内容物中，另一方面又要能够抵御致病微生物体的入侵，这就需要在肠道内达到微妙的平衡，这部分内容将在第六章中进一步讨论。在消化道上部，由专门细胞分泌的胃酸是重要的抗菌防御机制。中和胃酸会使人体更容易被摄入的生物体感染。其他隐蔽的重要免疫防御机制则存在于其他消化道分泌物中，例如唾液、胆汁，以及大肠中的薄层黏液。

除了这些特定的结构外，所有细胞都具有识别何时被感染的机制（我们将在第二章中做进一步讨论）。这些机制会导致该细胞的死亡，从而使感染无法扩散；同时，分泌物也会释放出重要信号，抑制病毒和细菌的生长并警示和召集其他免疫细胞。

10

其中最重要的就是干扰素,我们会在第二章中做进一步讨论。

免疫系统中的特殊结构

除了上述的基本免疫机制外,免疫系统中更为复杂的活动具有自己的结构,不过这些结构呈散布状态(见图3)。**白细胞**(或者说白血球)是其中非常重要的细胞,它们和红细胞、血小板一样,由骨髓产生。白细胞亚群呈高度多样化,根据自身的特殊功能,可大致分为**骨髓白细胞**(在骨髓中发育)和**淋巴白细胞**(在淋巴结构中发育)。淋巴结构包括胸腺、淋巴结和脾脏。我们将在第二章中进一步讨论骨髓白细胞,不过简单来说,骨髓白细胞在完全成熟后会离开骨髓并在体内游走,一旦发现感染或组织损伤,它们都能随时随地做出免疫反应。相比之下,许多淋巴白细胞需要先接受一段时间的"教育";而且,尽管淋巴白细胞也可以对整个身体进行有效的检查,但就长期来看,它们总是在特定的组织中发挥作用。

胸腺位于胸部中央、胸骨后方;实际上,在进行胸腔外科手术时,为了打开胸骨进入胸骨后方组织,医生有时会移除胸腺。胸腺在儿童时期最为重要,这与免疫系统的主要发展时期一致,不过到了后期,胸腺开始萎缩,在个体成年及进入老年时,胸腺已经被脂肪组织所替代。T细胞需要在胸腺中进行发育。实际上,"T细胞"这个名称中的T就是胸腺英文名称的首字母,表示来自胸腺;而相应地,B细胞是在鸟类的法氏囊和哺乳动物的骨髓中发育的,"B细胞"这个名称中的B就是法氏囊和骨髓英文名称的首字母。在第三章中,我们将进一步探讨胸腺内部发生的"教育"过程,而胸腺的重要性也可以通过未能形成胸腺后的

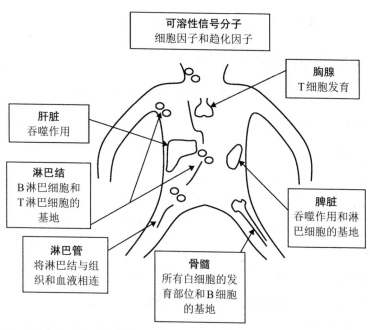

图3　许多免疫解剖结构对于免疫系统的发育和正常功能的发挥至关重要

巨大影响来进行评估。从胚胎学上说，胸腺起源于**鳃弓**。鳃弓
是一种位于颈部的鳃状结构，从进化学上来说十分古老，鳃弓也
可以发育成内耳和下颚。在某些具有先天性缺陷的个体中（例
如，迪乔治综合征），这些鳃弓无法正常发育，这意味着婴儿出生
时就没有胸腺，因此缺乏形成T细胞的合适区域，这就使他们极
易发生感染。但有趣的是，现在可以通过胸腺移植进行治疗（在
皮下插入胸腺组织），这样就可以支持T细胞的发育，从而降低
12 感染风险。

　　任何组织中都存在T细胞和B细胞，但是它们最开始来自
淋巴组织。淋巴结存在于身体的不同部位，例如，在颈部、腋窝
和腹股沟处都存在明显的较小的球状活动结构。通过利用特殊

的细胞表面受体并响应淋巴结自身释放的化学信号，淋巴细胞能够通过特定的小静脉进入淋巴结。已在骨髓和胸腺中成熟但尚未受到特定感染的淋巴细胞（即，**幼稚**淋巴细胞）通常会长期驻留在淋巴器官中。同样的，那些对感染做出反应并形成长期记忆的细胞（请参见第四章）也将返回到淋巴器官中。因此，在包括人类在内的多种不同动物中，淋巴结在启动和维持免疫反应方面具有重要的作用。例如，缺乏生成淋巴结信号的小鼠（例如，经基因工程改造使小鼠的淋巴毒素受体基因发生突变）就会出现严重的免疫缺陷。

正如前文所述，淋巴结由血液供养，不过淋巴结还有另外一种重要的输入物——淋巴液。淋巴液是一种体液，通常由人体组织产生，通过细窄的静脉状结构运输。淋巴液可以看作血液中血浆的**滤液**——受人体循环系统的压力从血管中排出，但不含红细胞。淋巴液为免疫系统提供了关于组织状态的重要信息来源，将细胞和蛋白质携带至淋巴结进行采样，并在必要时快速启动免疫反应。淋巴液的流量不仅对淋巴结的功能至关重要，而且对于控制体液平衡处于正常状态也十分重要。在淋巴管受损的情况下，例如，由蠕虫感染引起的丝虫病，或是通过手术或放射疗法治疗癌症后，长时间的淋巴积液会导致肢体肿胀：这种情况被称为**淋巴水肿**。

13

一方面淋巴结不断地对淋巴液和人体组织进行检查，而另一方面脾脏则为淋巴细胞的发育提供了另一个重要场所，同时也对人体的整个血流进行监视。脾脏位于腹部左侧，藏在肋骨下方，在过去人们对它认识不足，并不认为它是一种免疫器官。然而，脾脏在摄取细菌和清除感染方面起着主要作用。这在缺乏脾脏的人体中——例如，腹部受伤后需要通过外科手术将其切除——表现十分明显。这类人群极易被特定的细菌感染（特别是像那些具有荚膜的肺炎球菌），因此需要接种疫苗，通常情况下还需要使用预防性抗生素，从而在最大程度上降低暴发性感染的风险。这种清除功能不是由淋巴细胞完成的，而是由被称为**吞噬细胞**（即，吃细菌的细胞）的特殊髓系细胞（**巨噬细胞**）来完成的，这些吞噬细胞可以吞食在脾脏中缓慢流动的血源性细菌。因此，在诸如疟疾之类的慢性或复发性感染中，脾脏的体积会大大增加。

吞噬细胞活性十分重要的另一个主要部位是肝脏。在肝脏中，被称为**库普弗细胞**的特殊巨噬细胞，会把经肠道流出的静脉血中的细菌清除干净，从而提供了进一步防御。

然而，尽管上述这些结构很重要，但仅凭这些结构来描述免疫系统就会遗漏很重要的一点：免疫系统具有高度关联性和整合性，包含许多肉眼不可见的可溶性成分。前文已经讨论了主要的免疫细胞类型（骨髓细胞和淋巴细胞），它们通过利用一系列它们能够分泌并感知的信号分子进行沟通从而发挥功能。被称为**细胞因子**的可溶性信号分子，会提供有关免疫反应细胞应如何做出反应的信息；这些细胞因子是影响增长的信号；细胞因子也可以作为效应分子来增强抗病毒防御能力（例如干扰素，请参见第二章）。

趋化因子是一组特殊的可溶性化学物质，可以帮助免疫细胞进行定位，例如将免疫细胞引导至淋巴器官或感染部位。这些小分子通常由一种细胞分泌，并在受到感染的组织中形成一个梯度来吸引所需的免疫细胞。为了调节免疫系统出现故障的

14

情况，我们正在研究用于分别抑制这些分子的复杂方法，因此对这类具备免疫信息的可溶性传导分子的了解也变得越来越重要。

完全不具备物理结构的**补体系统**，是免疫系统具有完善性的方面之一，关于补体系统的内容我们将在第二章中做进一步讨论。补体系统不仅提供了可以识别微生物体和组织损伤的一种机制，而且也提供了一种直接反应的机制，例如，与细菌结合并杀死细菌。

因此，可以认为整个身体就是一个免疫系统——体内的每个细胞都具有其自身的内部免疫反应机制，而器官中则具有专门的结构来抑制感染。通过对这些细胞反应的监测和整合，可以形成一支更为"专业"的免疫细胞队伍，它们具有用于细胞"教育"和发育的特定结构，并且在这两者之间，一系列可溶性介体和游离细胞之间一直保持着沟通。

免疫系统被称为"漂浮的大脑"，把免疫系统与神经系统类比是十分恰当的。因为免疫系统和神经系统都需要对各种内部及外部的信息做出反应，并且这两个系统除了遵循预设的行为规范外还需要进行"学习"。在神经系统中，个体与生俱来的（即，先天性）行为与习得性行为的差异是显而易见的（先天性行为，例如呼吸、对疼痛的反应；习得性行为，例如语言能力、音乐和运动技能）。这些活动由大脑的不同部位负责。

这种现象也广泛地存在于免疫系统中。与生俱来的先天免疫反应可以立刻对一般的感染做出有效反应。这与**适应性**免疫反应联系紧密，适应性免疫反应包含针对个体感染的习得性和特异性反应。先天免疫是指初始的免疫反应，可以保护个体免

15

受直接威胁。适应性免疫系统则更为复杂,特异性更强,对于首次出现的威胁需要更长的反应时间;但是,适应性免疫系统具有像大脑一样的记忆力,这种记忆力的产生是由于特定的感染对于淋巴细胞(记忆B细胞和记忆T细胞)的诱导。在第二章中,我们将探讨如何触发免疫系统的最初反应,以及免疫系统如何拥有与大脑相似的感知力。

第一反应者：先天免疫反应

每一次免疫反应都会从某个地方开始，可是免疫系统如何知道何时做出反应呢？这个重要的问题已经困扰免疫学家们长达数十年之久，因为这对于理解免疫系统的正常反应（例如，针对感染）和异常反应（例如，在自身免疫性疾病中）以及设计疫苗、研究针对癌症和传染病的新疗法都至关重要。在本章中，我们将研究如何启动免疫系统，以及这些初始的相互作用有多重要。

多年来，免疫系统的中心范式是其区分自身与非自身的能力。换句话说，自身所含有的东西不会引起任何反应，而外来物质的存在（例如，移植的器官）则会触发反应。关注点就在于免疫系统如何识别抗原，即由生物分子（例如，蛋白质）衍生的特殊结构。不过，在过去二十五年中，人类的认知得到了发展，可以明显地看到：不只是抗原本身，暴露抗原的环境也十分重要。在20世纪90年代，波莉·马青格提出了**危险理论**：如果出现一种新的抗原，当有标明它是危险的额外信号存在时，就会引发功能性免疫反应。

17

机体如何感知危险的这一发现，也带来了这一领域的重大突破；早在几年前，查尔斯（查理）·詹韦就提出了免疫系统对病原体相关分子模式（PAMP）非常敏感这一观点。这些PAMP是可以预测的微生物体共有的特征，但与它们的宿主不同。此类受体的多种家族已经进化到可对病原体进行"感知"，这一发现充分证实了詹韦的理论，从而为这一领域带来了突破。对这类PAMP的精调识别可以启动宿主对特定病原体的防御，从而推动免疫反应的后续进程。

人们发现这一过程的涵盖面要广泛得多，包括损伤相关分子模式（DAMP）。这些信号存在于受损的组织中而非健康的组织中，例如，细胞损伤后细胞内的物质会释放到周围区域。PAMP和DAMP的感知的相关属性，解释了组织损伤和感染的情况都会出现相似的免疫反应的原因。

感知危险

并非所有细胞都具有感知PAMP的能力。就感知PAMP的能力这方面而言，即便是先天免疫系统中的特殊细胞，其中一些细胞亚群的感知能力也要大于另一些细胞亚群。这些细胞包括一种重要的髓系细胞（见图4）。**单核细胞**是大量存在于血液循环中的一种细胞亚型，可以迁移到组织中，然后在组织中转化成巨噬细胞，即我们在脾脏中遇到的吞噬细胞。单核细胞还可以转化成一种被称为**树突状细胞**的细胞；长期以来，人们都没有注意到树突状细胞，但是自树突状细胞被发现以来，它们就在免疫系统中占据着重要位置。如图4所示，树突状细胞表面呈内卷的波浪形（树突状细胞以前被称为**面纱细胞**），并且具有一系列

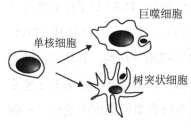
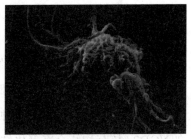

图4 隶属于髓系细胞的巨噬细胞和树突状细胞是吞噬细胞，它们来源于单核细胞，存在于血液循环中。电子显微照片中显示的是树突状细胞

PAMP感受器，所以它们可以识别遇到或摄取的特定分子。因此，这些细胞能够利用多种感受器来感知危险，而一旦感知到危险，就可以有效地协调从那一个节点开始的免疫反应。

细菌具有一系列可以被宿主细胞感知的常见PAMP。LPS（脂多糖）就是一个很好的例子，LPS是许多细菌——尤其是革兰氏阴性细菌——外表面膜的一部分。（在一个多世纪以前，汉斯·克里斯蒂安·革兰就发现了这些用于细菌分类的细菌染色剂，目前人们仍在使用这些染色剂。）即使在LPS的浓度极低的情况下，免疫系统也会通过Toll样受体（TLR；此处为TLR4）感知到LPS的存在。TLR4的激活是一种有效的危险信号，这种信号可以激活树突状细胞来分泌细胞因子，召集更多的免疫细胞，并启动一系列广泛的免疫反应。如果上述方法可以有效控制感染，那么LPS会消失，系统就会快速回到正常状态。在细菌广为扩散的情况下，例如由**脑膜炎双球菌**引起的脓毒症，对LPS的反应会过度激活免疫系统，并带来具有危害性的后果。

LPS并非人体可以感知的唯一的微生物产物。实际上，TLR4本身也能够识别由疟原虫产生的脂质。其他Toll样受体

19

可以感知细菌细胞壁的其他成分,例如,TLR2对于检测结核分枝杆菌(Mtb)十分重要,结核分枝杆菌会导致结核病(TB)。这些受体位于细胞表面,可以监测细胞外环境。其他类似的受体位于细胞内,监测吞食的或细胞内的PAMP(即,来源于感染细胞的生物体的PAMP)。一种不同类型的细胞内受体——例如NOD2(核苷酸结合寡聚化结构域蛋白2)——可以识别革兰氏阳性细菌的特定成分。NOD2之所以引起人们的关注,是因为编码该蛋白质的基因具有多态性,也就是说,NOD2的基因因人而异(第五章将对此进行详细探讨)。该基因的某些变异体可以对抗引起麻风病的**麻风分枝杆菌**。NOD2的一些变异也与炎症性肠病密切相关,可能是通过改变对肠道细菌的处理方式来实现的。人们认为,免疫系统中存在冗余或备份,庞大的感受器群能够应对不同的威胁(例如,NOD2本身可以感知病毒),但是,各种受体在抵御感染和疾病的发展过程中仍然可以发挥主导作用。

病毒利用细胞机制在它们所感染的细胞内进行复制,同时也会释放独特的危险信号。当RNA病毒(例如,流感病毒)进行复制时,它们会生成双链RNA,这是健康的宿主细胞没有的一种RNA形式。因此,在宿主中形成了许多警报系统来识别这些双链RNA(例如,利用蛋白质RIG-I进行识别的系统;见图2),而且与识别LPS的系统一样,它们的敏感性也很高。这种敏感性十分重要,因为通常情况下病毒的复制速度非常快,因此反应的灵敏度对于在宿主被大面积感染之前启动免疫反应至关重要。然而,某些病毒,如丙型肝炎病毒(HCV)已经进化出破坏该信号传递的机制,从而让自己处于优势地位。通过RIG-I可

以在受HCV感染的肝细胞中检测到来源于HCV的RNA，但是
HCV随后又产生了一种可以特异性地破坏信号传递的分子，从
而有效地阻止了抗病毒反应的启动。

危险的DNA也可以被感知。在人类DNA中，某些类型的
序列会通过被称为**甲基化作用**的过程进行化学修饰，而细菌中
这些相同类型的序列没有被修饰，因此它们可以被Toll样受体
TLR9识别，从而启动免疫反应。类似的，哺乳动物的DNA位于
细胞核内，而病毒的DNA位于细胞核外，因此这也可以被最新
发现的一种利用两种关键分子CGAS和STING的通路发现。感
受器CGAS通常以一系列游离的分子形态存在于细胞中，它们
本身是没有活性的。然而，如果出现外来的DNA，这些分子就
会和外来DNA结合在一起，形成一种多单位的酶，这种酶会产
生一种被称为环状GMP的小分子。随后，环状GMP会将信号
传递至STING，从而使细胞产生干扰素（见图2）。

免疫系统中存在这几种充当警铃的危险感知机制。总体而
言，它们被描述为先天机制，是一个健康机体的内在能动部分，
不需要事先接触过相关病原体就可以在必要时做出免疫反应
（见图5）。

对危险做出反应

在免疫系统收到警报之后，重要的是快速采取行动来抑制
病原体的扩散。人体可以立即启动许多反应，这也是先天免疫
的重要部分。总体来说，这些反应导致了人们长期以来所认为
的**炎症**，即为了应对组织损伤，被激活的细胞在组织中的局部
聚集。

21

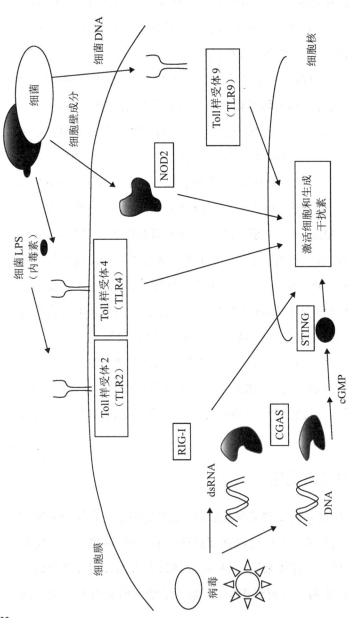

图5 感知危险的机制包括通过RIG-I感知细胞内双链RNA的识别，通过CGAS感知细胞质内的DNA，以及通过Toll样受体感知其他病毒配体和细菌细菌配体

一些重要的早期反应是由干扰素系统介导的。半个世纪前，人们发现了干扰素，它可以限制病毒的复制；并且随着时间的推移，干扰素在宿主防御中的核心作用得到了有力的证实。具有限制干扰素信号突变的动物对病毒高度易感。大多数细胞都可以产生I型干扰素（α和β），并且大多数细胞还具有这些I型干扰素分子的受体。干扰素α释放的信号，可以在细胞内诱导出一系列让人震惊的反应，同时可以对数百种基因进行上调。这包括可以抑制病毒复制的基因，例如，通过降解细胞内的RNA和抑制蛋白质的生成来实现。随着时间的推移，这些干扰素在指导适应性免疫反应和产生有效免疫力方面也起到了重要作用。

干扰素也可用于治疗，例如用于治疗慢性乙型肝炎病毒（HBV）和HCV。不过，干扰素对于HBV和HCV的治疗只是部分有效，因为这两种病毒已经适应了宿主体内天然的干扰素反应。而对于HCV，另一个不同的干扰素系统——干扰素λ——很重要。具有特殊的干扰素λ3基因的个体，在接触HCV后清除该病毒的概率要高出五倍，从而避免了慢性感染和肝脏疾病。

病毒寄生于细胞内部，因此控制病毒的机制主要集中在被感染的细胞上。相反，通常情况下细菌更多地是在细胞外进行复制，因此需要不同类型的免疫反应。其中之一就是引入一大批先天免疫细胞——**中性粒细胞**。中性粒细胞来源于骨髓，具有一个多叶核，细胞质中含有细小颗粒。中性粒细胞与**嗜酸性粒细胞**和**嗜碱性粒细胞**等相关细胞一起被称为**粒细胞**和多形核细胞或**多形体**。中性粒细胞在细菌和真菌的防御中非常重要，如果中性粒细胞缺失——例如，治疗癌症的药物会抑制

23 中性粒细胞在骨髓中的发育——会使个体处于受到严重细菌感染的高风险中。中性粒细胞通过吞噬微生物体（即，**吞噬作用**），生成来自过氧化氢（一种有效的生物漂白剂）衍生物的有毒介质，并释放含有抗菌分子的颗粒来发挥作用。吞噬作用是宿主防御中的关键步骤，一旦中性粒细胞吞噬了微生物体，细菌就会在含有高活性**溶酶体**的细胞中的专门区域通过消化的方式被破坏。

正常情况下，中性粒细胞的存活时间不长，只有几天；在针对感染的急性反应情况下，中性粒细胞会"战死沙场"。不过，在中性粒细胞"战死沙场"之前，它们会做出最后的"壮举"——挤出细胞核。这就会形成来自细胞核长链DNA的一个NET（中性粒细胞外诱捕网），它的形态与蜘蛛网十分相似，可以捕获细菌，提高细菌清除率。相关的粒细胞——嗜酸性粒细胞和嗜碱性粒细胞——参与的是不同类型的免疫反应，特别是由蠕虫感染引起的免疫反应。这些细胞与T细胞、驻留在组织中的**肥大细胞**一起参与上述免疫反应，关于这一内容，我们将在第六章中进一步讨论。

中性粒细胞的活动可能会损害宿主，因此需要通过指导让免疫反应集中在感染部位并组织其功能。其中一个重要的协调者就是**补体系统**。补体是免疫系统的重要组成部分，补体在肝脏中产生并在血液中循环。在这里，补体起到一个复杂的蛋白质团的作用，即所谓的**级联反应**：通过按顺序激活该家族的其他成员，一个小信号可以随着发展得到局部放大。补体级联反应可以通过诸如抗体结合等不同方式被首先激活。不过，补体级联反应也可以通过与微生物或先天性危险信号（例如，来自组织损伤）的直接接触而被激活，从而立即释放活性成分来结合细菌并吸引中性粒细胞。经过补体成分修饰或**受过调理作用**的细菌，更容易被吞噬细胞吞噬和破坏。其他补体成分可以与细菌结合并在其膜上形成孔状结构，从而破坏细菌。在此类"终端"补体蛋白存在缺陷的家族中，补体作为抗菌分子的特殊重要性是显而易见的——缺乏补体会导致入侵性细菌（例如，**脑膜炎双球菌**）的感染风险增加。

人类的补体系统是高度进化且复杂的，约有三十种蛋白质以严格调节的方式与先天免疫反应和适应性免疫反应有关（见图6）；而且，从进化的角度而言，补体系统本身非常古老，可能已经有五亿多年的历史了。补体成分存在于刺胞动物（例如，水母和海葵）中，补体系统在其宿主防御及炎症反应中发挥作用。

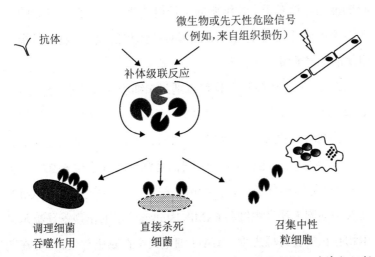

图6　补体蛋白可以被抗体、微生物或先天性危险信号（例如，来自组织损伤）激活。补体蛋白一旦被激活，就会发生"级联反应"，从而激活更多补体成分并大幅度放大信号

先天免疫反应不只有吞噬细胞的作用。淋巴细胞也可以通过自然杀伤（NK）细胞的活性来发挥作用。NK细胞来自骨髓，但不需要在胸腺中成熟；它们具有一组能够响应压力信号和病毒感染的受体。NK细胞可以通过释放有毒颗粒杀死细胞，或者释放干扰素从而抑制病毒复制。NK细胞还可以感知危险，它们拥有可以通过细胞表面的特殊压力信号的表达来触发的受体，还可以识别"失踪的自身"，即病毒为了进行掩藏而清除了细胞表面的蛋白质。

与NK细胞有关且最近才被发现的另一类淋巴细胞是**先天淋巴细胞**（ILCs），这是一种罕见但有效的免疫细胞亚群。NK细胞存在于组织中，在引发和控制炎症中起到重要作用。NK细胞能有效分泌细胞因子，因此可以指导许多其他细胞的效应器功能。肠道的有趣之处在于，它具备生成细胞因子白细胞介素22的能力。这对于上皮细胞的生长很重要，因此，此类细胞的激活不仅可以通过免疫反应来协调对病原体的反应，还可以指导组织的即时修复。

最后，先天免疫反应也可以通过T细胞和B细胞（尤其是T细胞）介导。直到最近才发现的具有高度丰富性的一组特别有意思的细胞，是**黏膜相关恒定T**（MAIT）细胞。这些细胞能够识别细菌PAMP，在这种情况下，它们是细菌合成维生素B2（核黄素）时产生的小分子。许多细菌和酵母菌都会产生细菌PAMP，而人类细胞无法产生细菌PAMP，因此该分子的出现就是提示微生物存在的良好标志物。MAIT细胞集中在黏膜部位，可以在宿主防御过程中提供预警和即时的效应器功能。MAIT细胞只是一种所谓的**"桥接"**种群，即一组同时具有先天免疫特征和适应

免疫系统

性免疫特征的细胞。

急性期反应

到目前为止，我们已经了解了对感染的第一反应所涉及的分子和细胞。就整个生物体而言，这些反应会被整合，不仅会产生局部效应（炎症），而且会引起生理上的重大变化（见图7）。分泌可溶性介质（例如，细胞因子、干扰素）意味着其作用可以遍布整个人体，因为这些信号分子可以产生远距离作用。例如，在对由细菌感染诱导的细胞因子产生反应时，肝脏会分泌几种有助于宿主免疫反应的蛋白质。肝脏会发出关闭铁储存库的信

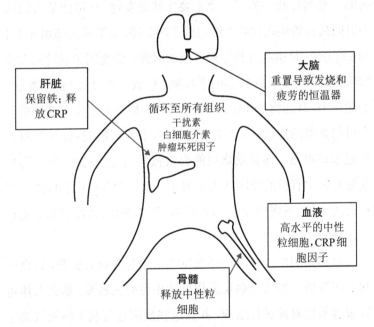

肝脏
保留铁；释放CRP

循环至所有组织
干扰素
白细胞介素
肿瘤坏死因子

大脑
重置导致发烧和疲劳的恒温器

血液
高水平的中性粒细胞，CRP细胞因子

骨髓
释放中性粒细胞

图7　对感染的急性期反应是由对危险的感知引起的，而且会导致遍及全身的多种作用，这些作用主要由处于循环中的干扰素和其他细胞因子等可溶性介质介导

号来限制细菌获得铁,而细菌需要铁才能进行复制。肝脏还会分泌一种被称为**C反应蛋白(CRP)**的分子,该分子可以像补体一样调理细菌的吞噬作用。测量血液中的CRP是衡量细菌感染的指标,该方法广泛应用于临床医学。临床上使用的类似方法是测量血液中(从骨髓中释放的)中性粒细胞计数,其在急性期反应中会显著上升,尤其是在细菌感染而非病毒感染中。

干扰素对人体有许多影响,包括食欲改变和产生疲劳感(即所谓的"疾病症状")。我们认为类似流感的许多症状实际上是由干扰素反应介导的,这在使用干扰素进行治疗的时候(例如,治疗病毒性肝炎)尤其明显,且这种副作用十分常见。与感染有关的一系列症状中的另一个重要症状是发烧,这可能是人们认识时间最长的疾病症状。细胞因子的分泌,尤其是白细胞介素1和6的分泌,是引起这种生理反应的原因。细胞因子通过向人体"恒温器"(位于大脑底部的下丘脑)释放局部介质(前列腺素)而起作用,从而将"恒温器"重置在一个较高的温度。这种重置会引起典型的症状:个体会感觉寒冷,甚至可能发抖,但是身体摸起来却很热。尽管发烧可能会增强某些免疫功能,但是为何发烧对宿主有益的原因却尚不明了。急性期反应也会伴随许多行为改变,而发烧也许会限制感染产生的整体影响,甚至限制宿主之间的传播。

对感染的生理性反应还包括心率增加和血管扩张,这会引起血压降低。如果这些反应程度适中且时间较短,那么人体可以很容易地对此进行适应,并且这些反应也有利于将氧气输送到组织。然而,某些更严重的感染会引起过度反应,降低的血压会导致生命危险,引起感染性休克。即使用抗生素治疗感染,细胞因子的级联反应也会持续维持这种异常的生理状态,这种情况下个体需要在重症监护室中得到额外的支持,以监测和调节血压水平以及肺和肾等器官的功能。

先天免疫反应被调节至可以感知非常微小的局部信号,因此可以尽早识别危险。然而,先天免疫反应的作用具有系统性:对骨髓的作用是释放更多的中性粒细胞(所谓的**紧急粒细胞生成**);对大脑的作用是改变行为和重置温度;对血管的作用是改变血液运输。因此,先天免疫反应同时囊括了免疫系统中的一些最微妙和最显著的特征。也许是由于这些公认的显著变化,先天免疫反应在过去通常被认为是相对简单且常规的,不过随着对先天免疫反应的了解日渐增多,其复杂性也日益显现。

这些免疫反应在感知病原体的过程中高度进化,当然,病原体也相应地通过进化来逃避免疫反应。利用人体的先天免疫反应是疫苗研制和免疫疗法的关键——疣(人类乳头瘤病毒)的一种有效疗法是 TLR7 激动剂乳膏,而用于治疗病毒性肝炎的可溶性 TLR 激动剂正在研究中。迄今为止,有一项研究表明,并非先天免疫反应在前而适应性免疫反应在后,多数情况下两者是同时起作用的。先天免疫反应通过适应性免疫反应得到增强(抗体激活补体并调理细菌的吞噬作用),而适应性免疫反应则会利用先天免疫反应的效应器(例如,T 细胞召集中性粒细胞和嗜酸性粒细胞)。这种持续的活性意味着阻断先天免疫反应在治疗慢性炎症性疾病中具有重大价值,因为在慢性炎症性疾病中,此类通路处于异常且持久的激活状态。我们将在第七章中进一步讨论这个想法。

适应性免疫：(非) 自身发现之旅

本章要解决的一个关键问题是，免疫系统如何应对众多的威胁，包括人类从未遇到过的病毒种类（例如，严重呼吸道感染疾病SARS和MERS Co-V）。免疫系统中这种内在的多样性可以通过分析适应性免疫反应，尤其是B淋巴细胞和T淋巴细胞上的受体如何组合在一起来进行解释。

B细胞和抗体

B细胞是在骨髓中发育并能够分泌抗体以提供免疫保护的淋巴细胞。抗体是高度专业化的蛋白质，可以结合特定的靶点（例如，细菌或病毒的外衣），这种靶点被称为**抗原**或**表位**。抗体完成结合之后，可以阻断感染（**中和**），激活补体系统，并被吞噬细胞摄取。如果抗原位于细胞表面（例如，被感染的细胞或癌细胞），则可能导致该细胞被杀死。人体可以产生各种抗体，且这种建立广泛抗体库的能力十分重要——抗体产生过程中的缺陷会让个体处于病毒和细菌感染以及罹患癌症的风险之中。这种其他基因一样被编码在基因组之中，但它们还是利用一些特殊的技巧来创造多样性。

抗体（或免疫球蛋白）基因不是作为一个单一单元存在的——如果抗体基因是作为单一单元存在的话，我们会遗传大量高度相关的基因，这样甚至会带来无法确保个体免受威胁的危险。因此，要做的是将较小的基因片段进行组合，每个基因片段本身都各不相同，而通过各种组合形成的基因可以产生更多的可能性（见图8）。每个抗体由两条链组成：一条重链和一条轻链，而正是这些链的组合提供了特异性，换句话说，就是结合一个单独靶点的特定能力，例如，结合今年的流感病毒毒株，但无法结合去年的流感病毒毒株。免疫球蛋白重链基因最具特

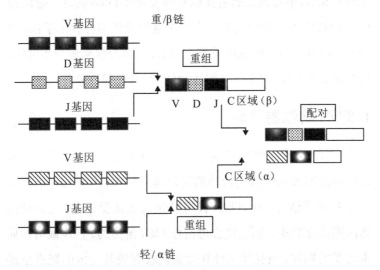

图8 抗原受体或抗体的DNA由重组的独立片段构成。这些片段表达为重链和轻链，并进行配对。除了α链和β链的使用不一样外，构建T细胞受体的过程类似

异性的片段，是在给定的 B 细胞基因组中由三种亚基——V、D 和 J——组合在一起的（**重组**）。这些亚基中的每一个都在基因组内并排多次出现（44V、27D 和 6J）。这些片段可以或多或少地随机组合，从而提供数千种产生抗体的潜在模板。实际上，由于组合连接过程中可能会引入其他核苷酸，因此多样性会更高（所谓的**连接多元化**），这可以进一步修饰关键位点的抗体结构。轻链上也发生了类似的过程，只不过缺少了 D 片段。实际上，人体中有两种不同的轻链基因，位于基因组的两个不同的位置。

每个 B 细胞都独立执行这一重组过程，因此，当数百万个 B 细胞生成时，它们可以充分探索重链和轻链组合的可能性，从而为宿主防御建立非常广泛的抗体库。B 细胞中的体细胞重组过程受到许多基因的严格调节，其中最重要的是 RAG（重组活化基因），RAG 小心地控制着操纵和修复宿主 DNA 的这一危险过程。RAG 的丢失会让宿主失去产生这种受体多样性的手段，因此也就没有了适应性免疫系统。此后，抗体会得到进一步修饰，从而提高有效性并"锁接"附加功能（请参见第四章）。

T 细胞：将细胞外翻

B 细胞会产生可以检测细胞外环境的抗体，因此可以在病毒感染细胞或在细胞间传播的时候捕获病毒，或者与生活在细胞外的细菌结合。B 细胞还具有特定的表面受体，这是一种抗体的膜结合形式。通过结合可溶性（即，游离的）抗原或诸如病毒之类的颗粒，该受体可使 B 细胞接收有关其受体的靶点呈递的信号。但是，病毒和其他病原体，包括一些寄生虫（例如，引 起疟疾的寄生虫）和细菌（例如，第二章中提到的导致结核病的

Mtb细菌）都生活在细胞内部，那么如何检测这种内部环境呢？这就要靠T细胞及其特定感应器：T细胞受体或TCR。T细胞利用与B细胞相似的原理在其细胞表面上形成受体，从而监测细胞的内部环境。

标准模型的T细胞受体的基本组成情况与B细胞受体非常相似（见图8）。该受体由一条α链和β链组成，具有与免疫球蛋白重链和轻链相似的基因，即V、D和J区域。

T细胞需要感知细胞内部的蛋白质，例如，在靶细胞内复制的病毒。为此，免疫系统已经发育出一条在细胞表面显示一个细胞的蛋白质内容物的通路（见图9）。所有细胞都具有通过**蛋白酶体**降解蛋白质的机制，该蛋白酶体是蛋白质切割酶的复合物，可形成桶状细胞器。通过严格调节过程中的一系列酶，靶向降解的蛋白质被一种所谓**泛素**的小分子所装饰。这包括入侵病毒产生的任何蛋白质。经过泛素标记的蛋白质被运送至蛋白酶体处，被切割成在十个氨基酸长度范围内的不同长度的短氨基酸序列——**肽段**或**表位**。这种肽段或多或少是随机产生的。其中一些肽段被主动泵入细胞的"出口仓室"——内质网——让一些专门的蛋白质将这些肽段"出口"至细胞表面。

为了达到这一目的，用于"出口"的蛋白质高度进化，且被编码至免疫系统的关键基因区域，该基因区域被称为**主要组织相容性复合体**（MHC），在人体中也被称为**人类白细胞抗原**（HLA）复合体，或者更常见的是被称为**组织类型**。HLA基因分为Ⅰ类和Ⅱ类两大类，在人体中Ⅰ类蛋白质分为三种主要类型：HLA-A、HLA-B和HLA-C。每一种分子都非常适合携带和呈递肽段，因为它们具有与细胞膜结合的柄状结构和一个含有一条

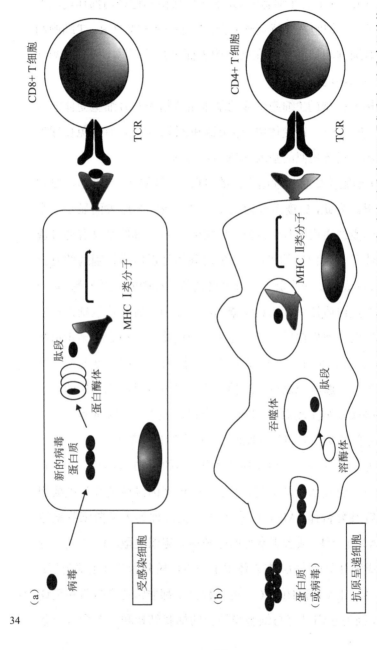

图 9 （例如来自病毒的）抗原 (a) 通过 MHC I 类通路呈递至 CD8+ T 细胞；(b) 则通过 MHC II 类通路，这是专门的抗原呈递细胞的特征

（图中文字）

CD8+ T 细胞
TCR
MHC I 类分子
肽段
蛋白酶体
新的病毒蛋白质
病毒
受感染细胞
(a)

CD4+ T 细胞
TCR
MHC II 类分子
吞噬体
肽段
溶酶体
蛋白质（或病毒）
抗原呈递细胞
(b)

凹槽结构的平台。肽段可以紧密地结合到该凹槽中。因此，一个满载的HLA分子在此凹槽中将含有一条与T细胞紧密结合且对T细胞"可见"的肽段。这些肽段可以通过受体被T细胞精确感知。

由于存在大量不同的病毒，因此也存在各种各样的肽段，所以通过MHC进行呈递的系统必须非常灵活。人体在进化过程中已经通过形成大量不同类型的HLA分子（**等位基因**）解决了这一问题。在全球范围内，人们已经发现人体中存在三千多种不同类型的HLA-A分子和四千多种HLA-B分子，这使HLA分子成为整个人类基因组最多样化的区域。与B细胞受体和T细胞受体不同，HLA分子不会重组，每个个体只会遗传六种这样的 I 类等位基因（从每个亲本处遗传一组HLA-A、HLA-B和HLA-C）。然而，HLA分子的多样性之高，组合可能性之多，以至几乎没有人具有完全相同的HLA分子。

由于HLA基因的高度多样性，导致了器官或骨髓移植中主要的匹配问题。因为在这种情况下，来自供体的不同HLA分子会被识别为外来分子，就像病毒一样，而且会诱导快速免疫反应（请参见第六章）。实际上，正是由于存在移植屏障这一特点，才首先吸引彼得·梅达沃等免疫学家把MHC作为一种"移植抗原"，而MHC在宿主防御中的作用直到20世纪70年代才由罗尔夫·辛克纳吉和彼得·多赫蒂阐明。HLA区域是人类基因组中进化作用最为明显的一个区域，其多样化程度最高。换句话说，形成广泛的HLA对我们作为物种的生存至关重要。可能是因为这最大限度地降低了微生物逃避T细胞反应并感染整个种群的机会。因此，寻找匹配的移植供体所面临的问题，正是成功防

35

御严重感染的进化策略的结果。

辅助性和杀伤性

能够响应结合在MHC I类分子凹槽中的肽段的T细胞,是I类限制性T细胞。这些细胞的另一个特征是次级受体CD8的表达。CD8不仅是这些细胞的有用标记,而且实际上还通过与MHC分子的微弱结合及稳定的相互作用增加了特异性。一旦CD8+ T细胞识别出受感染的细胞,就会被激活增殖(从而进行复制并放大反应),还会通过杀死靶细胞并释放许多信号分子对威胁做出迅速反应,因此它们被称为**杀伤性**或**细胞毒性**T细胞。

另一种主要类型的T细胞反应是参与协调免疫反应,即所谓的辅助性T细胞。这些T细胞的特征是其细胞表面CD4分子的表达,且会感知由MHC II类相关系统(该系统通常被称为"专业"抗原呈递细胞的免疫细胞亚群保存区)而非MHC I类系统呈递的分子。这些细胞中功能最强的就是树突状细胞,它具有非常强的摄取来自病原体的抗原并将其呈递给免疫系统的能力。树突状细胞及相关细胞(例如,巨噬细胞)可以摄取病毒、细菌或者此类病原体的一部分,并将其呈递至被称为吞噬体的专门仓室中。然后,吞噬体与被称为溶酶体的细胞器融合。溶酶体的内容物酸性很强,因此病原体被破坏并分解成肽段。随后,这些肽段立即被装载至II类分子上,被转运至细胞表面(见图9)。

因此,尽管B细胞能够感知并响应循环系统中的威胁(例如,整个病毒),CD8+ T细胞能够感知并响应细胞内的威胁(组织细胞中的病毒),但CD4+ T辅助性细胞可以感知由树突状细

36

胞等专业抗原呈递细胞提供的抗原。然而，尽管这看起来可能有些局限，但是CD4+ T细胞对于免疫系统的功能至关重要。这种重要性在艾滋病患者中得到了显著体现，因为受到HIV的靶向攻击，艾滋病患者中的CD4+ T细胞已经丢失。为何CD4+ T细胞如此重要，因为它们可以为CD8+ T细胞和B细胞提供帮助从而指导它们的活动。由于受到高度专业化的树突状细胞的指导，它们不仅能接收呈递的抗原信息，还会接收相关的其他信息。正如前文所述，树突状细胞还可以感知与特定感染相关的PAMP，并向CD4+ T细胞提供基本信号以指导其后续反应。由于这些指导出现在免疫反应最早期的阶段，因此CD4+ T细胞将负责随后的免疫反应。这种相互作用及其指导的Ⅱ类分子，对宿主免疫及其调节具有重要影响。辅助性T细胞的种类很多，其区别在于它们产生的细胞因子（例如，1型、2型和17型）不同。由于它们在宿主防御、自身免疫和过敏中起着重要作用，我将在后续章节中进行介绍。

非常规T细胞

其他具有不同目的的T细胞可以作用于细分领域。这些非常规T细胞不仅在发现抗原的方式上有所不同，在免疫反应中的作用也各不相同，因为通常情况下它们在血液中很少见，多存在于组织中。非常规T细胞还部分扮演了反应者的角色，请参见第二章。首先被发现的此类非常规T细胞是一个T细胞亚群，该细胞使用的不是α和β的TCR链，而是被称为γ和δ的一组类似的受体链，其靶点不是MHC。我们已经发现了一系列分子可以触发γδ T细胞，包括一种细菌的产物HMBPP（4-羟基-3-甲

37

基-2-丁烯基焦磷酸盐），其作为配体所起的作用非常强大。据报道，细胞表面分子嗜乳脂蛋白3A1充当了γδ细胞的呈递分子。γδ细胞在人体血液中相对罕见，但富集于肠道等的黏膜处，且会在细菌感染后扩增。γδ细胞在绵羊等其他哺乳动物中更为常见，且是主要的T细胞类型。

除了γδ T细胞之外，还存在非MHC特异性的αβ T细胞。顾名思义，恒定自然杀伤T细胞具有NK细胞的某些特征，但也含有TCR，尽管这些细胞来自胸腺且具有一致的独特α和β链。该受体能够结合被称为CD1d的MHC样分子，而该分子携带一个糖脂分子（即基于脂肪而非蛋白质的识别）。这些细胞所识别的一个重要分子是α半乳糖神经酰胺，它含有一个糖分子和一个来自细菌的脂类分子。在第二章中提到的MAIT细胞则给出了另一个例子，这些细胞识别MHC相关分子MR1而非MHC，呈

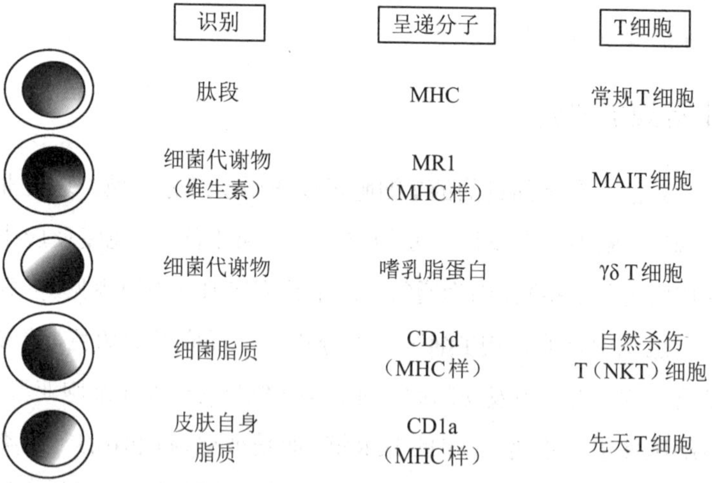

识别	呈递分子	T细胞
肽段	MHC	常规T细胞
细菌代谢物（维生素）	MR1（MHC样）	MAIT细胞
细菌代谢物	嗜乳脂蛋白	γδ T细胞
细菌脂质	CD1d（MHC样）	自然杀伤T（NKT）细胞
皮肤自身脂质	CD1a（MHC样）	先天T细胞

图10　越来越多的非常规T细胞亚群被发现可以识别不同类型的分子，其中一些分子与MHC分子相似但通常不具有多态性（即，个体之间并不相同）

免疫系统

递由细菌（而非人类）产生的维生素B2前体。这些非常规或非典型T细胞富集于人体肝脏和肠道上皮。可能还存在许多具有其他识别策略的T细胞类型有待发现，也许会为宿主，尤其是在屏障部位，提供防御（见图10）。

分布和再循环

通过该过程产生的淋巴细胞亚群并非在体内随机分布，而是在结构上精心组织的。这种情况对于快速启动免疫反应至关重要，我们将在第四章中进一步讨论。离开胸腺的CD4+和CD8+ T细胞的表面有一组受体，使其可以通过特殊通道进入淋巴器官。这是通过与组成所谓高内皮细胞微静脉这些组织中的血管内膜相互作用而实现的。相反，即使发炎或感染，它们也无法进入正常组织。肝脏是这一规则的唯一例外，因为肝脏的内皮具有间隙（**窗孔结构**或窗格结构），可以让**幼稚**细胞（即，尚未遇到病原体的细胞）和肝细胞群进行直接接触，这一特征可能与肝脏独特的免疫学相关（请参见第五章）。

幼稚T细胞存在于血液中，在淋巴结之间进行循环，并高度富集于淋巴结和脾脏中。幼稚B细胞同样集中于这些区域，这具有重要的生物学意义，因为幼稚B细胞需要与T细胞进行密切的相互作用从而变成能产生抗体的细胞。被激活的T细胞会离开淋巴结，在血液中循环，并在整个身体中重新定位或**归巢**于组织，从而提供局部防御能力。它们通过改变其细胞表面的受体来实现这一点，因此不再与高内皮细胞微静脉结合，而是被发炎的内皮吸引。前文提到的非常规T细胞通过已经形成的这种组织归巢程序进行发育，因此它们可以直接分布至组织中。这很容易理解，因为非常规T细胞的作用是提供即时保护，且它们不需要在淋巴结中接受进一步的"教育"和扩增。

淋巴管是淋巴细胞及其他免疫细胞重要的通行路径。淋巴细胞通过小淋巴管离开淋巴结，最终通过胸导管回流至血液系统。一旦回流至血液，幼稚细胞便可以重新通过循环回到淋巴结，确保B细胞受体和T细胞受体的整个范围在结构上均匀分布，从而应对各种威胁。

在本章中，我们了解了如何从每一种简单的方面来实现免疫系统的高度多样性。实现这一点的动力十分巨大，MHC是人类基因组中多样化程度最高的一部分，并在整个人类的进化过程中都承受着非常巨大的选择压力。一个群体中的MHC多样化程度越高，病原体攻击个体或整个群体免疫系统的可能性就越低，因为病原体必须重新应对每个个体。如果未能实现MHC的多样性将会是灾难性的，可能会让整个种群易受感染。

在B细胞和T细胞的抗原受体中，多样性的意义更为明显。该问题通过不同的进化方式得以解决，利用独特的重组方法从而有效地创造数百万额外的可能基因以实现这一目的。以B细胞为例，这些基因以及根据遗传模板生成的抗体会经过千锤百炼，从而可以对特定靶点呈现高度特异性。B细胞的基因组可以通过有效的"训练"以产生最佳的免疫反应。因此，第二章中提到的先天免疫反应的特征是敏感度和速度，而本章中讨论的适应性免疫反应的特征是多样性和特异性。在第四章中，我们将了解到应对此类威胁的免疫反应是如何协调的，以及如何充分利用潜在威胁的多样性。

40

41

制造记忆

到目前为止，我们已经了解了一般情况下免疫系统如何感知抗原（例如，通过PAMP和补体），以及如何特异性地靶向针对病原体（例如，通过B细胞分泌的抗体和T细胞上的TCR）。显然，所有这些都需要在空间上紧密协调，以便各司其职，但作用的时间也至关重要。让我们思考一下，暴露于病毒之后免疫反应是如何发展的，根据罗尔夫·辛克纳吉的信条：病毒是免疫学最好的老师。

启动免疫反应

为了制造有效的**记忆**，在感染的初始阶段，需要正确诱导或启动免疫反应。为了启动免疫反应，免疫系统必须采取的第一个步骤与激活先天免疫系统有关。如果没有这一步，就像用遗传缺陷小鼠进行的实验一样，适应性免疫反应在随后的许多情况下都会不堪重负。实际上，能在多数感染者体内引起慢性感染的HCV，可以抑制并逃避先天免疫反应长达数周之久，这样做

的目的是为了在感染者体内存活。入侵局部组织的病毒很快就会被巨噬细胞、树突状细胞等髓系细胞捕获，从而启动先天免疫

反应。通常，病毒会呈递多种PAMP，从而激活这些细胞并启动抗原呈递过程。

如果是为了让抗原呈递给各种幼稚T细胞，以期用合适的TCR将病原体与种类繁多的肽段进行匹配，那么启动这种过程的价值是有限的。树突状细胞需要重新定位至局部淋巴结，专注于T细胞集中的区域。此时会与公认的反应性T细胞进行一系列快速的相互作用，从而寻找可以匹配的条件，换句话说，就是一个可以识别其结合了MHC的肽段的T细胞。正如第三章中所述，MHC分子上存在的每个肽段上都可能含有TCR，尽管它们可能仅代表了正常T细胞池的百万分之一。因此，该过程必须十分高效，尤其是因为在这个节点上病毒已经开始快速复制，免疫反应的发展与其争分夺秒的竞赛也在进行当中。免疫反应的这一阶段被称为启动。

一旦带有合适TCR的T细胞得到认定，那么对于该T细胞的信号就会十分有效，且该细胞内将发生重大变化。要确保TCR本身保持不变，否则将失去反应的特异性。因此，为了通过该识别来放大反应，一旦接收到这样的信号，那么首先出现的反应就是细胞增殖，通过细胞分裂来产生子细胞。这种增殖反应是巨大的，在几天之内，对单个病毒肽段做出反应的T细胞可能会扩增至体内CD8+ T细胞总量的十分之一。这一过程十分有必要，因为T细胞需要检查身体中的每处组织，以寻找并破坏被病毒感染的细胞。T细胞内发生的变化也十分显著，除了增殖以外，T细胞快速获得了一些特性，例如，破坏抗原的能力；生成干

扰素γ（与干扰素α一样具有多种抗病毒特性）、肿瘤坏死因子、趋化因子等可溶性分子；吸引其他细胞。与感染前发现的幼稚细胞不同，这种细胞被称为效应性T细胞。此时，CD4+ T细胞被激活，抗病毒CD4+ T细胞群不断扩增。

同时，淋巴结也同样诱导了B细胞的反应。B细胞的这种反应在结构上是离散的——尽管B细胞只是位于局部位置，但B细胞分泌的抗体会对整个机体产生作用。B细胞需要CD4+ T细胞的帮助才能实现充分优化的抗体反应。这种反应集中在被称为**生发中心**（见图11）的淋巴组织的特殊区域。在抗原集中的部位，B细胞之间为了信号和空间相互竞争。这是一种非常有效的方法，可以确保最有效的抗体（来自所有可用的抗原）得到快速扩增。因此，在生发中心内，B细胞的增殖是经过精心协调的。

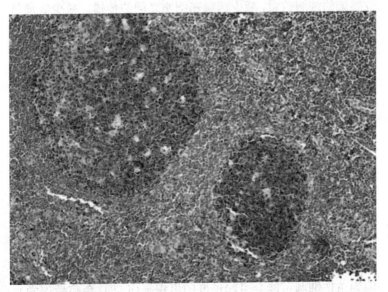

图11 B细胞的反应发生于生发中心。图中为扁桃体切片中不连续的深色结构

44

这种反应的结果是分泌抗体的B细胞激增并离开淋巴结，在发生感染后一周左右的时间，可在血液中检测到这种B细胞，且抗病毒抗体的数量迅速增加。值得注意的是，并非所有针对病毒蛋白的抗体都是相同的。尽管无法一直成功地中和靶点，但针对病毒包膜蛋白（该蛋白能让病毒附着并感染宿主细胞）的抗体通常具有最大的保护价值。如果病毒以其他方式（例如，通过补体）被结合并被免疫系统识别，这也可能提供某种保护。结合病毒并阻止其感染其他细胞的抗体被称为**中和抗体**。生成高水平的中和抗体是许多疫苗的策略目标，因为这可以提供针对感染的完全保护，即所谓的**消除性免疫**。

初始的先天免疫反应、由此产生的干扰素，以及后面快速出现的细胞（T细胞）和体液（B细胞/抗体）免疫反应，可以降低被感染的细胞数量，减少病毒在细胞之间的传播。减少病毒复制对免疫进化十分重要，因为这意味着降低抗原水平和触发先天免疫反应。此处，B细胞的反应和T细胞的反应出现了一些不同。B细胞会继续成熟并产生抗体，通常在人（感染之后）的余生中，在其循环系统中都可以检测出这些抗体。此类抗体由已迁移至骨髓并主动分泌抗体的B细胞产生，这些B细胞现已成为被称为**浆细胞**的专门细胞。相比之下，T细胞的寿命要短得多。如前所述，T细胞的反应迅速扩张，效应性CD8+ T细胞在血液和组织的含量很高。然而，在没有进一步刺激的情况下，这些细胞会迅速死亡，细胞数量急剧减少。这种动态的扩增和减少，在限制身体暴露于非常危险的杀伤细胞方面具有重要的意义，因为杀伤细胞可能会引起过度的组织损伤（即，**免疫病理学**）。然而，该细胞群不会完全消失，而是会作为一种免疫记忆而长期

45

持续存在。

形成免疫记忆

免疫记忆被认为是适应性免疫的特点。从某种程度上说，免疫记忆十分简单。实际上，关于免疫记忆的定义可以回溯至第一章中对于免疫的定义：免疫记忆可以防止个体再次暴露于同一感染。如果人体对抗原具有免疫记忆，则可以保护该个体免受潜在的致命感染。这种记忆反应可以起到广泛的作用，其原因是保护性介质（T细胞、B细胞、抗体）的含量较高，且具有与先前遇到的感染做斗争的合适品质。这些介质细胞既具有数量性又具有质量性，这就意味着它们可以快速做出反应，从而为个体提供免受感染的绝对保护，或者至少在感染形成或引起症状之前快速控制或清除感染。

由自然感染引起的免疫记忆最著名的一个例子，来自法罗群岛上一个与世隔绝的大西洋社区，该社区成员由于海员的到来而断断续续地暴露于新的感染。1846年，丹麦医生彼得·帕纳姆前往法罗群岛调查麻疹病毒的暴发，该病毒在未暴露过的人群中具有很高的发病率，在易感人群中具有很高的致死率（1911年暴发于太平洋岛屿罗图马岛的麻疹导致五分之一的儿童死亡）。帕纳姆指出，尽管致病率确实很高，但仍有一部分人未被感染，这些人是年龄较大的岛民，曾暴露于1781年的麻疹大流行并得以幸存。

所以说，形成于一个世纪以前的保护性免疫记忆一直延续到了下一个世纪。很容易想象这种毁灭性的传染病如何影响了免疫系统的进化（见图12）。

46

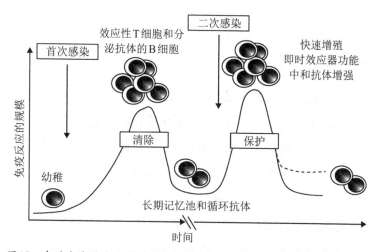

图12 在效应阶段后，B细胞和T细胞的数量减少，免疫记忆形成。当再次遇到相同的感染时，这些细胞将重新快速扩增，并在血液中达到更高的水平（被称为**免疫增强**）

　　这种长期的保护机制是什么呢？长期以来，免疫学家们对这个问题争论不休，同时这个问题也持续吸引着疫苗研究领域的极大兴趣。幸运的是，对于疫苗研究而言，研制有效的疫苗并不需要对这一过程有充分的了解，在多数情况下，只要利用身体对感染的自然反应就足够了。然而，对于复杂的感染（例如，HIV），假设把这一机制比作引擎，则需要在免疫记忆反应的引擎盖下进行寻找，拆开引擎并进行重新设计（请参见第七章）。

　　记忆反应中最容易理解且广义上说最有效的部分是B细胞47的诱导，以及持续数十年的强效抗体。随着时间的流逝，B细胞可以改善其抗体的质量（黏性或**亲和力**）。通过进一步调整感染最初几天内产生的原始免疫球蛋白的基因序列可以实现这一点（请参见第三章）。B细胞当然不知道如何改善其抗体，不过它采取了"热情试验者"的方法，尝试了所有可用的方法以找到更有效的抗体。该过程由B细胞特别使用的基因活化诱导胞嘧啶脱氨酶（AID）控制，该基因使其免疫球蛋白的相关区域产生突变。AID作用于现有的B细胞反应，有助于提高记忆反应的质量（亲和力或黏性），这被称为**亲和力成熟**。

记忆抗体反应被具有高度活性的IgG抗体所主导，该抗体具有一种额外的特殊品质，即可以穿过胎盘。这与生成的第一种IgM型抗体相反（IgM抗体是急性感染的良好标志物，可用于临床诊断）。诱导强效IgG抗体的一个重要结果是，母亲的记忆反应可以保护未出生的胎儿在子宫内免受感染。除此之外，它还具有足够的持久性，可以持续保护新生儿。在婴儿出生后的前几个月中，由母体转移的抗体水平会有所下降，但仍可以在婴儿最脆弱的时期提供有效的保护。这种附加的（也许是最重要的）好处是自然发生的，但也可以进一步加以利用。例如，当前正在测试的抗呼吸道合胞病毒（RSV）疫苗的一种十分有意思的接种方式是让孕妇接种疫苗。这种常见的疾病在低龄儿童中最为严重，提高母体的抗体水平可能是确保婴幼儿在最大风险期能够得到足够保护的一种简单方法。

B细胞记忆池分为两部分：一组是位于淋巴结中的**休眠**记忆细胞；一组是被称为浆细胞的高度分化的B细胞集合（前文已讨论过），这些浆细胞会回到骨髓并生成有效的抗体。这两种方式的结合提供了免疫系统内的平衡，从而使抗体介导的保护得以持续。循环特异性抗体可在中和病原体时提供即时保护，而且在某些情况下可以通过测量血液中的抗体水平来推测能否提供成功的保护（例如，在接种HBV疫苗后进行这种测试以确

48

保免疫反应已经实现)。然而,在接种疫苗之后,这些抗体的水平确实会随着时间的流逝而下降,但是可以通过激活B细胞记忆池来维持长期性的保护,一旦重新遇到该病毒B细胞会迅速增殖,产生更多的抗体分泌细胞,形成较高的抗体水平。这就意味着,即使在暴露于病毒数十年之后,该系统仍可以重启,快速分泌更多的抗体并提供有效的保护。

T细胞记忆及其分布

T细胞记忆有些复杂,因为它没有像抗体水平这样可以等同于**保护性免疫力**的简单标志物。尽管如此,我们还是了解被诱导的T细胞的记忆类型及其在宿主防御中可能的作用,大致与在B细胞中观察到的相似(对于杀伤性CD8+和辅助性CD4+ T细胞而言都是如此)(见图13)。因此,有一些T细胞变成了休

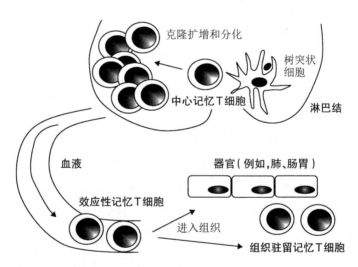

克隆扩增和分化

树突状细胞

中心记忆T细胞

淋巴结

血液

器官(例如,肺、肠胃)

效应性记忆T细胞

进入组织

组织驻留记忆T细胞

图13 淋巴结中富含中心记忆T细胞。血液中含有效应性记忆细胞,且富集于外周器官。另一组T细胞记忆细胞群被发现驻留于组织中

49

眠T细胞，在功能上并未被激活，但是当个体再次暴露于同一感染时会做出反应。这些T细胞位于淋巴结和脾脏内，如果它们呈递于抗原呈递细胞（例如，在启动阶段），那么淋巴结和脾脏就是重新遇到抗原的理想位置。

另一组T细胞的生活方式更为活跃，归巢于外周组织（例如，肝脏、肠胃、肺等），并维持效应器功能（CD8+ T细胞的杀伤性能力和特定细胞因子的即时分泌）的某些要素。

后一种细胞从许多方面来说都像是急性效应性细胞，被称为**效应性**记忆，与位于淋巴结中被称为**中心**记忆的休眠细胞相反。在对先前遇到的抗原做出反应时，中心记忆细胞将会增殖并获得效应器功能，再次归巢于组织，因此这两种细胞群并不彼此独立。在某些低水平的慢性感染（例如，CMV）中，病毒永远无法彻底清除，因此记忆池会不断被激活并伴随有这些细胞的增殖。最终的结果是，大量效应性记忆CD8+ T细胞逐渐积累，从而对单一的肽段做出反应，有时候甚至占据了血液中整个T细胞记忆群的大约三分之一（此过程被描述为**记忆膨胀**）。

除了这些定位差异之外，T细胞记忆群还可以通过其他方式实现多样化，从而有助于调整针对特定威胁的免疫反应。例如，人们最近发现，位于组织中的某些记忆T细胞群似乎已经永久地迁移至组织，即所谓的**驻留**记忆细胞。在完全驻留之前，这些细胞可能在组织感染的早期反应中起到特定作用。当然，总的来说，T细胞在组织防御中起着独特的作用，与B细胞通过分泌抗体从远程起作用不同，T细胞的即时出现和局部效应器功能，需要T细胞的直接存在和局部效应器功能来保护屏障表面。

50

其他T细胞已经形成了聚焦于生发中心的生活方式。T细胞在生发中心反应中的辅助作用,对于形成长期的B细胞记忆至关重要。疫苗学家已经学会通过将靶向目标附着在特定蛋白质,从而吸引并激活这些辅助细胞的方式来利用这一特性,即所谓的**结合**疫苗。针对肺炎球菌(**肺炎链球菌**是导致儿童和老人感染肺炎的主要原因)的新型疫苗非常有效,而制备这种疫苗的原理就是上述特性。T细胞的其他亚型也可以在此类具有特殊特性的反应过程中生成。其中包括与蠕虫防御及过敏相关的2型细胞,以及与细菌和酵母菌防御相关的17型细胞。这些内容将在第五章和第六章中进行讨论。

利用B细胞和T细胞的记忆进行免疫保护

在了解了记忆形成的机制之后,现在让我们来思考一下如何在当前的疫苗中利用这一机制,以及这些知识如何为未来的疫苗研制提供信息。经典的疫苗被称为**减毒活**疫苗,通常是已在组织培养物中生长并且在此过程中**毒性**减弱(即,致病能力降低)的病毒。牛痘疫苗是爱德华·詹纳用于预防天花的第一种疫苗,它是一种与天花有关但感染牛群的病毒。牛痘病毒能感染人类,但引起的疾病症状更温和,病程更有限。由于此类疫苗是基于病毒研制的,因此它们会诱导一种与真实感染相似的反应:识别先天免疫反应的触发因素,呈递抗原,诱导B细胞和T细胞对呈递的抗原做出反应,随之形成长期记忆。如果疫苗和真实病原体的抗原相同或基本相同,就可以诱导广泛的保护性反应。这确实是一个很容易产生长期有效免疫力的理想状态,甚至可能由于病原体是活的而会在特定环境中维持微量的水平,从而足以在长时间内微妙地增强免疫反应。这类疫苗为许多人预防了麻疹、流感和小儿麻痹症等的感染,疫苗接种也已经根除了天花(见图14)。

另一种简单的方法是使用蛋白质抗原。例如,这种方法在诱导针对**破伤风梭菌**(一种发现于土壤中的微生物,会感染伤口,导致破伤风)毒素做出反应方面发挥了很好的作用。在这种情况下不需要针对细菌的抗体,只需用蛋白质中和有害毒素即可。破伤风类毒素的给药方式,是通过简单的处理使蛋白质毒素失活并变得无害,然后诱导生成有效的抗体,从而阻断这种高效毒素的活性。类似的疫苗方法可以抵抗**白喉杆菌**(引起白喉的细菌)毒素。20世纪20年代,拉蒙和德孔贝分别研制了破伤风疫苗和白喉疫苗,这两种疫苗在近一个世纪内几乎维持原样,并在这段时间里挽救了无数生命。

52

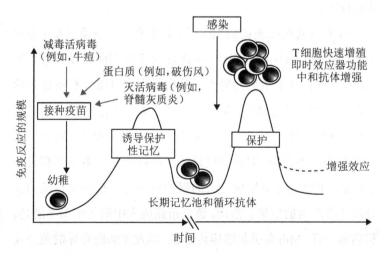

图14 该图显示了与感染之后记忆形成的相同过程,不过在这种情况下,这一过程是由疫苗诱导的。记忆T细胞和B细胞也会出现相同的诱导过程,一旦遇到真正的感染时就会发挥相同的保护作用

蛋白质抗原通常与**佐剂**一起使用，佐剂是一种可以引起非特异性炎症从而增强免疫力的物质。常用的一种佐剂是明矾（铝盐），可以激活多种先天免疫反应的通路。不过，也许将来可以通过运用关于完全启动B细胞和T细胞所必需的通路的新知识，来得到经过专门设计的佐剂。通常，它们也需要得到免疫增强，因为清除蛋白质十分容易，并且需要反复的暴露，从而通过扩增、亲和力成熟和类别转换所需的发生于生发中心的反应来驱动B细胞。同样，由于抗体水平趋于下降，并且需要更多的记忆池和浆细胞来维持这种水平，因此这类疫苗通常需要在此后一段时间间隔后进行免疫增强。然而，尽管存在这些局限，基于蛋白质的疫苗在诱导抗体方面依然十分有效。将灭活的整个病毒作为疫苗也取得了类似的进展，例如，路易·巴斯德研制的狂犬病疫苗可以彻底保护人类免受狂犬病这一致命疾病的侵害。

由于生活在细胞内的Mtb（请参见第二章及第三章）等细菌不受抗体或B细胞的影响，因此针对这种细菌的疫苗很难研制，但也存在几个主要的靶点。其中最古老且唯一获得许可的疫苗是BCG，它是Mtb的减毒活疫苗，而全球已有约二十亿人感染了Mtb。由巴斯德研究所研发的BCG（卡介苗）敲除了其基因组的重要部分，因此高度减活。该疫苗在许多国家都进行了试验，可以为儿童提供有效的保护——儿童罹患这种疾病会导致非常严重的后果。然而，该疫苗在成人中的效用尚不清楚。和病毒一样，Mtb会引起细胞内感染，因此T细胞介导的免疫反应对清除Mtb非常重要。血液中某种特定抗体的水平代表一种保护性功能，然而与抗体不同的是，确定抗Mbt的保护性免疫水

免
疫
系
统

53

平，以及在众多蛋白质中筛选出最佳靶点并不容易。由于Mtb与人类都能接触到的无害分枝杆菌拥有相同的抗原，且该分枝杆菌在后期可能会影响人体对BCG（或新型疫苗）的反应，因此这项任务变得更为艰巨。

免疫记忆造福人类的一种用途是，将免疫力从一个人转移到另一个人身上，即所谓的**被动免疫**。它指的是抗体从母体转移至婴儿的这种自然情况，不过也可以将抗体提纯或浓缩从而应用于临床。这种治疗方式的一个例子是，将缺乏诱导自身免疫球蛋白能力的个体所丧失的记忆替换掉。定期向这些个体输入具有广泛特异性的免疫球蛋白，可以保护这些人免受严重感染。这种被动免疫的方式在许多特定的情况下已被医生使用了多年，例如，强效抗血清可以用于保护不具备免疫力但已暴露于HBV、水痘（在受到免疫抑制或怀孕的情况下）或狂犬病的个体。被动免疫的方式也可以用于被蛇咬伤之后来中和毒液。研制具有单一特异性、高度靶向性的单克隆抗体，在这一领域具有巨大的潜力（另请参见第七章）。

在这种情况下，记忆的概念一直吸引着免疫学家和神经科学家。在这两种情况下，一个事件的长期"烙印"是通过复杂的多单元系统形成的，该系统不会在单个部位存储或检索信息。即使有可能识别出我们标记为"记忆"的淋巴细胞，它们也只是更庞大团队中的一部分。在这两种情况下，演练的一个要素是修复系统中的记忆——反复的抗原刺激或长期感染，会对塑造记忆状态产生巨大的影响。在这两种情况下，有可能产生错误的记忆，这是免疫系统中交叉反应的自然副产品。在第六章中，我们会讨论自身免疫中错误记忆所带来

54

的后果。通过接种疫苗事先形成记忆，或者用英国雄狮队橄榄球教练的话说就是"首先发动报复"，已经挽救了自詹纳时代以来的无数生命，而在未来面对新型传染病威胁时有可能拯救更多生命。

免疫力过低：免疫失败

免疫系统功能良好的时候，我们大多数时间都不会注意到它其实一直在工作。然而，它是持续有效的，从而防止寄生在个体皮肤及肠道内的微生物体造成严重的感染，同时也抑制多数人自婴儿时期就感染的慢性病毒。然而，在某些个体中或在某些条件下，免疫反应可能会失败，这就会导致严重的疾病，具体会引起哪一种疾病，则要根据确切的失败机制而定。在本章中，我们将探讨这种失败是如何发生的，特别是基因变化和HIV感染所引起的免疫失败，同时我们也可以从中了解到正常免疫系统的工作原理。

冗余、多态性和敲除

免疫系统是由多个部分组成的复杂机器。在理想的情况下，每个部分功能良好，可以诱导针对共生细菌的适当水平的免疫力（即，无需太多）和抵抗传染性威胁的强大防御力（即，足够）。如果某些方面出现故障，则可能会产生许多结果，就像汽车零件出现故障会产生不同的影响一样。一个较为合理的结果是，什么也没有发生。因为对于这样关键的系统，显然存在某种内置的冗余。例如，人体含有多种形式的干扰素α，且承担的作用基本相似（即，保护细胞免受病毒感染）。HIV的关键入侵受体之一是被称为CCR5的分子，该分子是一种趋化因子受体，可为T细胞提供运输方面的信息。尽管该分子广泛存在，但是CCR5的遗传缺陷对宿主的健康影响很小，不过它对HIV感染会产生巨大的影响，稍后我们将会探讨这一点。丢失某些分子可能类似于失去备用轮胎——只要其他四个轮胎还正常工作，就不会引起注意。

其他基因缺陷会产生巨大的影响。所谓的**通用γ链**对于淋巴细胞生长和存活所必需的许多分子的信号传导至关重要，它的丢失会导致重症联合免疫缺陷。在这种情况下，多数淋巴细胞亚群根本无法正常发育，被感染的个体受到高度免疫抑制。在第一章中，我们讨论过一种病例：在罹患迪乔治综合征的个体中，胸腺无法发育，从而导致了T细胞免疫的灾难性失败。这种缺陷相当于汽车油箱中出现了一个大孔，即使其余的部分完好无损，汽车也无法运转。

免疫系统中还存在许多其他缺陷，或者说个体之间存在细微差异（基因多态性），这对于免疫防御具有更为具体的影响。特定先天信号基因的丢失会导致对小范围感染的敏感性（例如，大脑中罕见的病毒感染）。一组特定干扰素基因（干扰素λ3和λ4）的突变，会影响HCV的清除率，以及对治疗的反应，但显然影响很小。再拿汽车做类比，这种情况就像是丢失了后视镜，大多数时间不会引起注意，但是会存在一个影响特定操作的特定

免疫系统

盲点。这些特殊的关系令人特别感兴趣,因为这可以告诉我们很多让个体免受感染性威胁所需的特定要求,以及免疫系统如何进化以应对这些威胁。

考虑到个体之间的差异可能会影响免疫反应的质量(被称为基因**多态性**的微小差异),人类基因组中最重要的区域是MHC,它决定组织类型或HLA类型(见图15)。正如第三章中所述,这些分子负责将由病原体衍生的肽段呈递给T细胞上的TCR。实际上,只有可以将病毒的肽段结合到MHC分子凹槽中的那些部分,才对细胞免疫系统可见——T细胞或多或少对其他部分视而不见。这就好像MHC分子需要揭示病毒提供的信息,而其余的信息则是隐藏信息。

MHC是人类基因组中多样化程度最高的部分,长期以来MHC经历了严格的筛选,从而导致了人类群体中MHC分子的

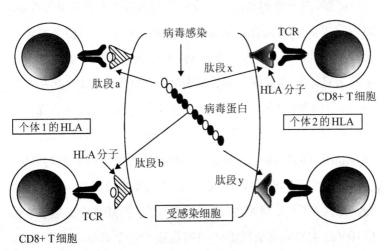

图15 个体1具有一组HLA分子,一旦被一种病毒感染,可能会呈递肽段a和肽段b;而个体2将呈递肽段x和肽段y。实际上,同一种病毒在这两个个体的免疫系统"看来"是不同的

多样性。因此，就选择呈递的肽段而言，个体之间的MHC分子差异很大，这可能会对其引起的免疫反应产生很大的影响。换句话说，尽管两个人可能同时感染了完全相同的病毒，但他们呈递给T细胞的肽段可能完全不同。在某些情况下，这可能没有任何区别，所有T细胞的反应可能都一样好。但是，在其他情况下，选择正确的肽段就十分重要。在HIV和HCV等慢性病毒感染中尤其如此。在这种情况下，肽段的选择可能至关重要。某些MHC分子将免疫反应集中在更有效的病毒靶点区域，从而为T细胞提供了相对的优势。那些天生就有这种有利的遗传特点的个体，在感染之后会出现更好的预后（请参见本章后文中讨论的HIV）。同样的，由于病毒肽段的靶点具有高度可变性，或者甚至是缺少这种靶点，某些不利的MHC类型指导的免疫反应效果较差。

　　显然，对一系列肽段产生反应的能力对个人而言至关重要，因为它提供了找到合适病毒靶点的最大机会。在整个群体中具有多样性的选择也是一种优势，通常情况下病毒就无法通过适应来逃避免疫反应。有数据表明，伴侣的选择（包括在人类中）可以由源自此类MHC分子的嗅觉信号驱动，因此选择那些不同的MHC类型会让后代获得不同MHC分子的数量最大化。但并非所有动物都如此幸运，在MHC选择非常有限的鸡群中，马立克氏病等病毒已成功适应了宿主的免疫反应来增强其感染力。在人类中，尽管MHC的多样性很高，但是我们仍然观察到像HIV之类的病毒会随着时间的推移在整个群体中实现适应，从而逃避了MHC以及T细胞的识别。据说，MHC分子以这种方式在病毒上留下了"足迹"，但同样的，病毒也通过如此密集的选择在MHC上留下了"足迹"。

MHC及其所呈递的肽段对免疫反应至关重要，因此MHC（或HLA）的类型与多种疾病相关（包括自身免疫性疾病，请参见第六章内容）。然而，这不是个例，即使范围比较窄，人类遗传特性中的自然变异也会导致免疫反应减弱或增强。另一个重要的例子是，在HCV感染中可以确定干扰素λ区域周围的自然变异与感染的预后密切相关。在感染这种病毒的情况下，由于存在有效的免疫反应，一些个体可以自发清除感染。如果干扰素λ区域出现特定的突变，那么该比例就会增加约四到五倍，并且还增加了治疗后成功清除病毒的概率。

干扰素λ是干扰素的亚型，与前文提到的干扰素α和干扰素β具有许多相同的抗感染特性，但干扰素λ活动的组织范围更为有限，主要是在肺和肝脏等组织中起作用。实际上，保护性基因类型在某些人群中非常普遍，因此可以推测存在某种选择性的作用力驱动了这种情况——尽管至今尚不清楚它是否会影响其他感染。这也许是"后视镜"基因的一种案例：对免疫系统实现最佳功能至关重要，但仅在相当特殊的情况下才重要。

免疫系统的先天性错误

某些基因改变会导致特定基因的缺失——"敲除"。这可能对人类免疫系统产生相当精确的影响（见图16）。尽管此类突变很少见，但可以揭示特定通路在控制某些感染中的关键作用。一个典型的例子就是17型通路的缺失，从而揭示了该通路对控制真菌感染的关键作用。携带影响此通路的突变的个

60

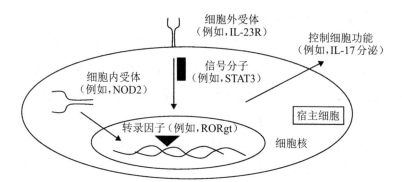

图16　宿主防御系统的缺陷可由细胞表面受体、信号分子、转录因子或效应分子的突变而引起。诸如TLR和NOD2之类的识别分子会影响免疫激活中的早期事件

体,例如,细胞外受体IL-23R、信号分子STAT3、主调节转录因子RORgt(利用17型通路控制细胞)中的突变,或控制细胞功能(例如,IL-17分泌)的基因中的突变,会遭受反复和持续的真菌感染。但这并不意味着17型通路仅与真菌防御有关——实验表明,它显然也与细菌防御有关。不过,确实可以表明17型通路在真菌防御中的作用是独一无二的,不能通过其他通路来实现。

　　与人类免疫反应相关的人类基因数据非常有价值,但也非常罕见。在过去的几十年中,人们通过分析特定缺陷的小鼠模型,从而在这方面的研究中取得了巨大进展。小鼠的免疫系统已经得到了充分的研究,且现有许多方法来检验小鼠对感染、肿瘤和其他疾病的反应。为了研究特定分子的作用,可以通过将基因缺陷靶向精确地引入小鼠体内来进行研究。对于确定在正常免疫系统或防御特定危险中的特定分子、通路或者细胞类型的作用,这是一种尤为强大的技术。

尽管分子生物学的进展已经发现了许多影响免疫系统的缺陷的基础，但许多所谓的**原发性**（即，先天性）免疫缺陷仍有待进一步确定。有一种相对常见的人群（大约五万人中会出现一个）被称为**常见变异型免疫缺陷**（CVID）人群。这些个体显示出了一系列缺陷，其中多数缺陷会影响形成有效抗体反应的能力。由于制备抗体的路径很长，涉及抗原周围的 B 细胞和 T 细胞的协同作用，因此许多影响细胞功能和存活率的不同缺陷可以导致相同的结果。对于那些受影响的人，他们很容易受到感染，最明显的是肺部的细菌感染。控制不善的反复感染可以导致破坏性肺损伤（**支气管扩张**），其本身可能严重影响正常的免疫防御系统。

该临床表现确实指出了抗体在控制人体携带的常见微生物体（例如，**肺炎链球菌**）中的关键作用。肠道、泌尿道和眼睛等其他部位也会受到影响，这些部位可能会定期或连续地与细菌接触。此外，免疫失调可能与自身免疫现象有关，这表明了在正常情况下免疫系统的精细程度。但幸运的是，一旦诊断出这种疾病（通常并不能直截了当诊断出这种疾病，因为疾病的发展需要一段时间），向患者输送健康供体的免疫球蛋白就可以防御这种疾病的传染性并发症。由于免疫球蛋白水平下降且其半衰期约为三周，因此在没有基因治疗的情况下，这种疗法具有常规性和终身性。通过每种情况下潜在原因更好的分子定义，也许可以研究出修复特定缺陷的方法。

营养不良和免疫缺陷

在全球范围内以及整个人类历史上，免疫缺陷的一个重要原因就是营养不良。这可能有多种形式,包括某些特定微量营养素的缺失(例如,维生素和矿物质)以及蛋白质-热量营养不良,这些情况可能同时存在。这种营养不良的确切影响是一种可变情况,取决于分子的功能,例如,维生素D参与调节性T细胞的发育,而维生素A通路在引起黏膜防御的信号中起作用。T细胞含有与饥饿有关的激素受体。瘦素是一种重要的饱腹感激素(即,一种抑制食欲的激素),不仅可以作用于大脑,还可以抑制T细胞的功能,为饥饿(瘦素水平高)和免疫功能障碍提供了一种可能的联系。这是一个复杂的领域,可能会有多种不同的影响相互重叠,全球流行的蠕虫感染可以直接影响免疫系统(请参见第六章)和营养状况并引起铁的丢失,这些都可能影响对其他微生物体感染的反应。

HIV和获得性免疫缺陷综合征(AIDS)

病原体如何利用正常的免疫系统?一种方法是关闭免疫系统,大多数病毒都使用这种方法来争取病毒自我复制所需的特定部位和窗口时间。有一种病毒已经进化出一种策略,可以利用免疫系统,把它变成自己的优势,从而达到摧毁宿主免疫系统的效果。HIV-1(以及主要发现于西非的流行程度较差的近亲HIV-2)与许多发现于非洲灵长类动物(包括黑猩猩)身上的病毒有关。该病毒可能在20世纪中叶跨物种传播给了人类。像许多跨物种传播的病毒一样,该病毒在每一种新宿主中引起的疾病大相径庭。因此,HIV的亲缘病毒(所谓的猴免疫缺陷病毒或SIV)可以相对无害地存在于某些猴类体内。这可能是一种共同进化的过程,病毒已经适应宿主从而限制了病理过程,此外宿

63

免疫系统

主群体也已经通过进化来抵御感染。但是，在HIV跨物种传染时不再适用上述规则，HIV-1不仅逃避了人类的免疫系统，而且还摧毁了它（见图17）。

HIV-1破坏免疫系统的第一个理由是其靶向感染的细胞。HIV-1利用两种分子进入细胞，即CD4和一种趋化因子受体，通常为CCR5。CD4是标记T辅助性细胞的主要分子，它是用于T细胞受体识别MHC Ⅱ类分子的共受体。CCR5是一种受体，允许T细胞在其他细胞以趋化因子尾迹的形式出现后归巢于感染或发炎的部位。因此，通过使用这种受体，该病毒能够靶向针对T辅助细胞，特别是刚刚被激活的细胞。感染此类细胞可导致一系列结果，但这些结果对于宿主均不利。细胞可能会受到有效感染并产生更多病毒。它可能会被免疫反应识别并被CD8+ T细胞破坏。否则，病毒可能会进行整合并形成潜在形式，以便日后重新激活。

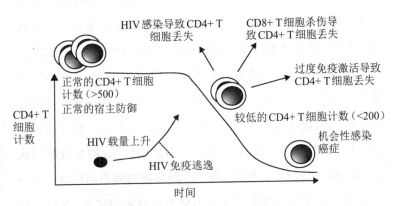

图17　CD4+ T细胞的正常水平大于每微升血液500个细胞，但是这一水平会随着HIV感染的进程而下降，而这又与病毒载量的上升有关。当低于每微升血液200个细胞时，宿主就存在极高的机会性感染风险

潜伏期的发展是HIV所属病毒组的一个特殊特征，即所谓的逆转录病毒。之所以被称为逆转录病毒，是因为虽然它们是RNA病毒，但是可以通过一种被称为**逆转录酶**的特异性酶将自身复制成为DNA。病毒的这种DNA形式是稳定的，该DNA是用于复制病毒基因组并实现病毒功能所需的所有蛋白质的模板。通过一种特异性**整合**酶把病毒插入宿主的遗传物质中，就可以把这种DNA整合至宿主基因组中。如果病毒具有活性，就会产生病毒蛋白，则该细胞将会成为CD8+ T细胞的靶点。但是，如果病毒是沉寂的，则免疫系统将对它视而不见，只要该细胞（或该细胞的后代）活着，该病毒就可以持续存在。这种特性使得病毒很难被完全清除。

如果CD4+ T细胞自身受到感染从而导致这类细胞的大量损失，这就是对免疫系统的一种巨大羞辱；但如果其存活时间较短，那么这类细胞很可能会迅速恢复。HIV的根本问题是其持续感染的能力，因此对免疫系统会产生长期而广泛的影响。HIV如何实现这一目标？前文已经提到的一个特点是发育一个潜藏地。然而，尽管从长期来看，这代表着清除方面的实际问题，但持久性的产生与血液中较高的病毒水平有关，因此在面临宿主免疫时会发生主动复制。通过分析宿主内病毒的进化并观察对单个宿主的快速适应，可以找到上述问题的答案。通过逆转录酶进行的HIV复制机制有一个非常有趣的缺陷，即新复制的病毒无法得到"校对"。因此，每一个新复制的病毒都包含至少一个突变。由于每天都会产生数万亿个新复制的病毒，而每个病毒的基因组包含大约一万个碱基对，这意味着该病毒产生的每个突变都可能为其所用。如此庞大的变异池为达尔文选择提供

65

了丰富的资源，这正是在面对B细胞和T细胞攻击时所观察到的现象。

HIV的抗体靶点位于病毒包膜中，由于它被高度**糖基化**（即，被糖分子包裹），因此这一靶点很难接近，该糖分子起着屏蔽作用。某些最重要和最脆弱的区域也被深深隐藏，只有在与细胞接触的时候才会打开，从而使病毒进入细胞内。尽管如此，仍可以生成针对HIV的有效抗体，该抗体能够中和并阻止特定病毒的感染。但是，病毒基因组中的单个突变可以很容易地保护病毒免受此类抗体的侵袭，而在包膜中形成的此类突变也可以在整个感染过程中观察到。换句话说，免疫系统能够通过产生抗体来有效控制任何特定的病毒株，但是病毒会先发制人，形成新的毒株，因此突变对病毒产生的代价很小。

所谓的**广谱中和抗体**（bNAB），换句话说，就是可以中和一系列范围很广的HIV突变体从而保护个体免受感染的一种抗体，它是HIV研究领域中的圣杯。实际上，在感染HIV后确实会形成这些抗体，但是所需的时间很长。如果可以使用简单的疫苗接种方法（例如，从一开始就将免疫反应聚焦于特定的靶点）来产生这些抗体，那么这将是该领域的巨大突破。

然而，该病毒也受到来自CD8+ T细胞反应的攻击，此外，产生突变的能力也使该病毒具有优势。某些MHC类型（例如，HLA-B27和HLA-B57）与发生HIV感染后产生的较好预后相关。极少数携带HIV的患者能够将其抑制到极低的水平，从而不会逐渐丢失CD4+ T细胞。这些所谓的精英控制者高度丰富了某些HLA类型，例如HLA-B27和HLA-B57（尽管还涉及其他因素）。这些分子结合病毒Gag蛋白中的肽段，病毒Gag蛋白是

66

一种将病毒基因组包裹在病毒中的分子。与病毒包膜相比，Gag 的突变能力相对受到限制，因此如果病毒被迫突变以逃避T细胞的识别，则可能对其Gag蛋白在适应性方面产生影响。也就是说，所形成的每个突变都可能对蛋白质作用的方式产生微妙的影响，从而损害病毒的复制能力，即所谓的**适合度代价**。

病毒管理这种平衡行为的一种方法是进行多个突变，以找到逃避识别的方法，同时限制适合度代价。因此，在这样的精英控制者中，病毒被有效地限制在一个角落，且在突变体方面，病毒的选择范围非常有限，并且已经对适合度产生了一些损害。然而，这种结果相对罕见。对于感染HIV的普通人而言，该病毒能够使其T细胞表位发生突变，以逃避CD8+ T细胞的反应并进行有效复制。

其他因素也可以限制抗病毒反应的影响，并且使HIV不仅可以持续存在，而且可以通过复制达到更高水平。一种因素是抗病毒免疫反应的特异性下调，被称为耗竭。此过程发生在免疫反应持续时间较长的情况下，并伴有负向开关或检查点的上调。其中最著名的是PD-1（程序性死亡受体1），当它与靶点PD-1配体结合时能够限制T细胞的功能。在长期的HIV感染中，这种过程确实十分活跃，与耗竭表型相关的一系列检查点分子的表达，是与病毒控制的失败相联系的。在LCMV（淋巴细胞性脉络丛脑膜炎病毒）的小鼠模型中，在持续感染期间会发生类似的过程，对PD-1的阻断可以恢复T细胞的反应，并与病毒控制相关联。这种方法是治疗传染病的潜在方法，不过对于癌症治疗会产生更大的影响。最终，"耗竭"的T细胞群只会丢失或被删除。在HIV中，尚不清楚T细胞反应真正耗竭到何种程度，但是对于限制CD8+ T细胞有效清除被感染靶点的能力的免疫反应的任何调节，都会微妙地改变各方面的平衡，从而有利于细胞内的病原体。

尽管免疫逃逸和免疫耗竭对于HIV的持续存在起着重要作用，但这并不能完全解释HIV中CD4+ T细胞大量丢失的原因。只有相对较小的一部分CD4+ T细胞受到了病毒的感染，但可以看到的是整个细胞群都受到了这种影响。对于这种放大作用的一种解释是**免疫活化**的形成：被激活的T细胞表达了某些表面标记（例如，HLA II类分子），从而可对这些T细胞进行跟踪。长期以来，人们发现HIV中普通的免疫活化会提示较差的预后。活化的免疫细胞可能会经历更为快速的更新和死亡，并且也更容易感染HIV。

关于为何会出现免疫活化的一种流行理论是，在感染早期，肠道中的CD4+ T细胞被大量感染。通常情况下，这些细胞在屏障防御中起着重要作用，失去这种屏障可能会导致细菌从肠道到血液的极低度迁移（所谓的**细菌易位**）。尽管这不足以引起严重感染，但足以激活免疫系统中的先天性感受器并触发T细胞的活化。因此，肠道中极早期的T细胞感染的长期后果，可能是通过这种非常间接的机制造成的，尽管针对病毒本身的其他先天反应也会起到作用。与这个论点相关的是，对于携带SIV 68却未对机体产生伤害的猴类（例如，乌白眉猴），其体内的这种免疫活化的水平非常低，但是携带的病毒水平却非常高。

因此，HIV感染会通过直接感染、免疫介导的杀伤、免疫活化的间接作用，以及其他许多可能的机制导致CD4+ T细胞的丢失。HIV还可以感染组织中的巨噬细胞（表达低水平的CD4）

和树突状细胞，也可以通过间接作用导致其他类型细胞（例如，MAIT细胞）的耗竭。然而，其中的血液中CD4+ T细胞计数是衡量感染发展情况，以及患者罹患该疾病风险的最佳方法。血液中CD4+ T细胞计数越低，个体对多种病原体的易感性就越大，而许多病原体的致病都具有所谓的**机会性**。

即使健康的人也容易感染TB，但是抵御TB需要完整的细胞免疫反应，这就意味着甚至是在相对较早的时期，罹患疾病的风险也会显著增加。相反，正常免疫系统中从未见过的许多相关的分枝杆菌感染，在CD4+ T细胞计数水平变低时就会变得十分常见。在这种低水平计数（每微升少于200个细胞，而正常水平是每微升大于500个细胞）的情况下，患者容易受到一系列机会性感染，包括由细胞内原生动物寄生虫（例如，引起脑损伤的**弓形虫**）、肠道病原体（例如，引起腹泻的**隐孢子虫**）、酵母和真菌（例如，引起肺炎的**肺孢子虫**），以及会对脑组织造成毁灭性破坏的JC病毒等引起的感染。这些都是一个健康的免疫系统可以轻松应对的微生物体，但很显然，这些严重的疾病表明了CD4+ T细胞在协调该系统时所起的持续作用。

在这种患有获得性免疫缺陷的患者身上出现的另一种疾病类型就是癌症。我们见到的两种主要癌症——卡波西肉瘤和B细胞淋巴瘤——是由不同的病毒引起的，分别为HHV-8和爱泼斯坦-巴尔病毒（EBV）。这两种病毒都来自同一个组别，通常在健康个体中很难清除（EBV是一种非常常见的感染），但是这些病毒通常都受到良好的控制，长期来看对人体无害。不受控制的复制与正常细胞向癌细胞的转化有关，因此，这种由病毒引起的癌症，是CD4+ T细胞在控制正常宿主对常见抗原的防御中发挥核心作用的另一个实例。

HIV是一种灾难性感染，而且由于本章中已经讨论过的原因，目前仍缺乏有效的疫苗。然而，药物治疗在抑制病毒复制和阻止疾病发展方面非常有效。CD4+ T细胞计数的恢复，在很大程度上与免疫功能的恢复，以及预防机会性感染和癌症有关。然而，该治疗仅具有抑制性，因此必须终身接受治疗。目前仅有一例完全治愈的病例。该病例通过骨髓移植来治疗血液癌，而移植的骨髓来自CCR5分子发生突变的供体。这种突变相对常见，并且可以影响自然感染率，如果此人含有两份这种突变基因，这将让他们对HIV具有高度抵抗力。接受移植的受体能够通过捐赠的骨髓有效地获得这种状态，因此没有接受进一步治疗就清除了病毒。但不幸的是，到目前为止，此人是这种治疗方式下的唯一治愈者。

这是一种不同寻常且激烈的治疗方法，但人们正在尝试各种方法，将HIV从体内的长期存储池中清除出去，并提供有效的治疗。正如前文所述，形成潜伏池的能力为病毒提供了优于宿主的有利条件，因为免疫系统不具备可视化的能力，无法对未出现病毒复制的细胞做出反应，同样的，药物也没有活性。有一种方式是使用多种方法激活病毒，然后在病毒继续传播之前摧毁已经暴露出病毒的细胞。这是一个复杂的领域，由于存储池在细胞中的实际位置、它们的状态，以及完全清除病毒的方法都很难确定。因此，目前最重要的方面是使需要接受治疗的人尽可能多地接受有效治疗，并且通过"教育"和适当干预（包括暴露前治疗方案）的方式来阻止感染的扩散。同时，寻找有效的HIV疫苗的工作仍在继续。

70

71

免疫力过高：
自身免疫性疾病与过敏性疾病

到目前为止，本书的大部分重点都放在针对微生物体的防御方面，这正是免疫系统进化的主要动力。这一点从免疫系统出现缺陷时发生的重症综合征就可以明显看出来（请参见第五章）。然而，考虑到引起组织损伤和炎症的能力，每一个免疫反应都必须进行适当且专门的调整。适当调整的失败会导致一系列免疫系统疾病，考虑到西方人口中健康状况和重大感染性疾病状况的整体向好，免疫系统疾病的重要性日益显现。在本章中，我们将讨论免疫系统如何关闭不需要的反应，以及在这个功能失效时会出现什么问题。这不仅包括研究典型的自身免疫性疾病，还包括出现过度炎症反应的其他疾病。它还包括对过敏性疾病的研究，过敏性疾病中会出现由特定免疫方式主导的对无害抗原的过度反应。

胸腺的耐受性

要了解自身免疫性疾病是如何发生的，重要的是要了解免疫系统如何采取措施避免这种情况的发生，即所谓**免疫耐受性**。

对于T细胞和B细胞而言，规则有所不同，但是由于CD4+ T细胞对于大多数长期抗体反应的形成至关重要，因此如果T细胞 受到良好控制，那么B细胞仓室就会随之形成。T细胞主要在胸腺中接受"教育"，因此这是习得自身耐受性最关键的部位。

　　T细胞的难题之一是如何确保生成的TCR有用。由于T细胞随机地把TCR放在一起，而抗原的识别完全依赖于该个体中存在的MHC分子，因此许多TCR在免疫反应中很可能没有价值。但对于B细胞而言，情况并非如此，因为B细胞的抗原非常宽泛，包括蛋白质、糖分子、脂质（脂肪），甚至是化学制品。问题的解决方式是为胸腺中的T细胞提供一些早期"教育"。胸腺中会发生两个基本过程，即所谓的**正相选择**和**负相选择**（见图18）。正相选择是一种确保存储池有识别自身MHC能力的过程，换句话说，就是该个体中存在一组特殊的MHC分子。

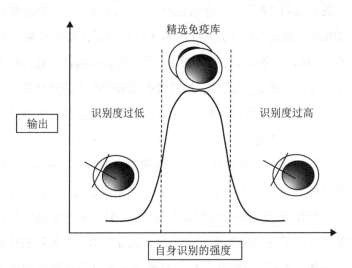

图18　T细胞（CD4+ 或 CD8+）在胸腺中发育时会遇到自身抗原。那些出现过强或过弱相互作用的T细胞会被清除（即，中心耐受性）

非常早期的、不成熟的T细胞一旦进入胸腺，就开始排列其T细胞受体。正如我们在第三章中讨论的那样，可用的排列方式有很多；而所需要的是能够与个体自身的MHC分子结合但不对自身产生反应的受体。这是一种有趣的平衡行为，因为在发育中的胎儿或新生儿的胸腺中没有可以利用的病原体，来为自体和非自体的选择提供基础。免疫系统解决此问题的方法是，通过被称为AIRE的特定基因的活性在胸腺中呈现多种自体肽段。这使胸腺中的细胞能够生成通常仅在体内非常特殊的细胞中才能产生的蛋白质（例如，来自胰腺或大脑），然后清除与这些蛋白质反应的T细胞。同样的，完全不能与自身MHC结合的T细胞也会被清除。只有那些在狭窄的"金发女孩范围"识别的细胞——数量足够但并不多——才能离开胸腺并形成幼稚细胞池。

这是免疫"教育"中非常关键的一步，AIRE基因的遗传缺失的影响，以及由自体反应T细胞和抗体诱导的疾病证实了这一点。AIRE是高度专业化的分子，可使胸腺细胞表达通常仅表达于特定组织的分子，例如，通常仅在胰腺中产生的胰岛素。因此，由于突变而导致的AIRE丢失，会使一系列原本会被清除的T细胞从胸腺逃逸，从而使个体（非常罕见）容易发生自身免疫性疾病。特别是，他们会遭受增强的对自身腺体（例如，甲状腺和甲状旁腺）产生的反应。作为一个明显的悖论，他们还可能会遭受增强的对酵母菌感染的易感性，但这是由于抗体与自身的细胞因子白细胞介素17产生反应而导致的。正如我们在第五章中所了解的，白细胞介素17在防御表面念珠菌感染中至关重要，因此自身免疫性疾病和免疫缺陷是缺乏自身耐受性这一

74

相同过程的结果。

外周耐受性

然而，即使AIRE功能齐全，该过程仍不足以完全防御自身免疫性疾病，因此免疫系统采取了"双重保障"的方法。例如，如果变异T细胞在没有经过适当"教育"的情况下逃离了胸腺，或者病原体和自体蛋白之间非常相似，则有可能破坏耐受性。这听起来似乎不太可能，但其实T细胞受体所识别的是一条短肽，该短肽结合在MHC凹槽中，并且可能只能呈递出两到三个可被识别的主要氨基酸。因此，即使病毒和大脑蛋白之间的肽段各不相同，但当它们结合并呈递至MHC中时，被识别的整个形状也可能会有所重合。因此，胸腺系统必须足够灵活，才能让T细胞逃离可能存在这种交叉反应的地方，否则对病原体的反应能力将受到极大限制。换句话说，它是有些漏洞的，或者免疫系统需要承担一些小小的风险来释放T细胞。

但是，如果变异（或潜在变异）T细胞在我们体内循环，为什么不是每个人都会患上自身免疫性疾病呢？其中的一种可能性就是忽视。如果抗原被隐藏起来，从而无法经过抗原呈递细胞（例如，树突状细胞）呈递给免疫系统（通过第三章中描述的过程进行呈递），就永远不会触发免疫反应。这种现象可能是由于缺乏对特定组织（例如，大脑）的反应性而导致的，大脑组织受到血脑屏障的保护；血脑屏障是一种物理屏障，能在很大程度上阻止免疫系统的细胞进入大脑。然而，在实验模型中，仍然可以通过接种脑源性蛋白质或肽段来诱导针对大脑的自身性反应。这种由外周诱导的细胞可以穿透脑部并引起疾病，因此这种"马

75

其诺防线"风格的防御不足以提供全面的保护。

组织也会进行自我保护。某些组织具有下调T细胞的机制，例如，它们可能会表达死亡受体（Fas-配体），该受体会与T细胞上的分子结合来杀死它们。前文中我们在免疫耗竭的情况下讨论过的PD-1，也是T细胞的重要关闭信号。缺乏PD-1的小鼠极易发生自身免疫性疾病。这是一个非常有趣的例子，病毒实际上利用了免疫系统中存在的关闭开关来下调免疫反应并使自身持续存在。另一种类似的抑制分子被称为CTLA4。CTLA4表达于T细胞上，并与被称为CD28的活化受体结合相同的分子。在免疫反应的启动中，CD28的触发作用非常重要，但是CTLA4可以干扰这种情况并消除这种反应性。导致CTLA4缺失的突变，会引起严重的自身免疫性疾病，并伴有淋巴细胞的明显增殖。有趣的是，CTLA4在人群中拥有许多变异体，某些变异体与肝脏、甲状腺、胰腺（会引起糖尿病）和肠道的自身免疫性疾病密切相关。这些变异体被认为可以调节宿主的免疫反应性，并且与其他类似的细微缺陷结合后会导致临床自身免疫性综合征的发展。

正如我们在第五章中了解到的那样，罕见的遗传疾病可以很好地说明特定细胞或通路的重要性，而IPEX综合征就是一个很好的例子。罹患IPEX综合征的患者体内丢失了FOXP3，这是对被称为调节性T细胞或**调节细胞**的一组T细胞的发育至关重要的分子。调节细胞的丢失与严重的自身免疫性疾病相关，这些细胞显然在维持我们健康、稳定的状态中起着重要的作用。调节细胞可以通过多种途径获得，并具有一系列特异性，但它们都能够对其他免疫细胞（尤其是其他T细胞）产生作用，从而抑制其增殖和许多其他功能。实际上，某些调节细胞来源于胸腺，无须删除自体反应细胞，胸腺通过诱导调节性程序可以使这些细胞得到很好的利用。这些调节细胞离开胸腺，可通过释放抑制性细胞因子，例如白细胞介素10和组织生长因子β（TGFb），来控制自体反应。它们还会表达高水平的白细胞介素2（IL-2）受体CD25，该分子被用作此类细胞的重要表面标志物。即使在较低水平，白细胞介素2也会被调节细胞识别并使其功能得到增强。当自体反应T细胞被激活时，就会产生IL-2，这可以增强调节细胞活性并限制自身免疫性疾病。

鉴于在胸腺中按顺序选择T细胞的方式，如果针对特定靶点产生了自体反应T细胞，就会相应地产生调节细胞从而监视周围的自体反应T细胞。但是，如果需要的话，调节细胞也可以经由其他的标准T细胞在外周进行诱导，这些细胞也会通过FOXP3的表达、调节活性的发展、IL-2受体的上调而发育成熟。然而，情况可能有些复杂。根据其来源，T细胞可能同时具有促炎性和调节活性。尽管这对于试图整齐地划分细胞类型的免疫学家来说有些困惑，但是对于系统来说，具有足够的可塑性，从而使T细胞能够随着情况的发展而调节其功能，显然是一种优势。

另一需要考虑的耐受性的进一步机制来自波莉·马青格的**危险理论**，或是查尔斯·詹韦的传染性非自身模型。这两个理论都认为，关于针对抗原免疫反应的重要问题不是自身与非自身的问题，而是如何将其呈递给免疫系统的问题。在炎症或感染（即处于危险情况下）中出现的抗原将会诱导反应，但是，在没有此类信号的情况下出现的相同抗原则不会诱导反应。数十年来，免疫学家仅凭直觉就了解了这一点，因为他们已经使用佐剂（通常是细菌产物）来诱导疫苗的有效反应。正如我们在第二章中所讨论的那样，这在分子层面是有意义的，因为我们对免疫系统如何感知此类危险信号或PAMP，以及它们对抗原呈递细胞的影响有了更多的了解。考虑到我们现在已经了解到胸腺中的自身耐受性过程是不完善的，因此还必须提供其他许多保护层，这也是有道理的。自身免疫性疾病的一个有趣但罕见的原因是，在疾病艾卡迪-古蒂耶综合征中表现出先天性免疫功能异常。患有这种疾病的个体无法有效分解DNA，所以当细胞自然死亡时，它们的DNA无法得到适当的处理。细胞内的游离DNA通过模式识别受体CGAS（请参见第二章）被识别为危险信号，因此这种遗传缺陷会导致高水平的先天免疫反应，就像是正在发生病毒感染一样。持续的炎症会在被感染的人群中引起自身免疫性疾病、组织损伤并导致严重残疾。

一个重要的信息是，在由病原体或炎症导致先天性信号缺失的情况下，无论是自身抗原还是非自身抗原，都应被忽略。这是一个很重要的情况，例如，如果其抗原通过树突状细胞从局部组织呈递至淋巴结，位于淋巴结中的自体反应T细胞就可以很好地通过TCR接收信号。如果树突状细胞没有接收到有关感染或炎症的任何信号，则该信号是安全的，其结果是一种被称为**无反应性**的现象，即失去了对进一步刺激的反应性。无反应性会导致无法对进一步的信号产生反应，以及只接收没有共同刺激或细胞因子的TCR信号的结果。这是一种非常有效的方法，可以十分精确地控制外周的自体反应细胞。仅向T细胞提供部分信号也是病原体的绝招。例如，HBV和HCV会诱导形成微弱的

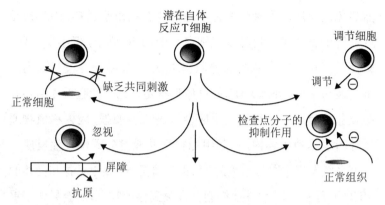

图19　许多不同且重叠的机制可能会导致对来自胸腺的潜在自体反应T细胞的功能性抑制或物理性清除（即，外周耐受性）

先天免疫反应，因此，尽管有大量抗原呈递给免疫系统，却无法 78
正确启动反应，并且可能需要数月的时间来诱导有效的T细胞
反应。图19总结了与外周耐受性有关的机制。

特定器官的耐受性：肝脏和胎盘

前文提到的HBV和HCV病毒也具有针对肝脏的独特特征，
而且由于它们的免疫学特征与其他组织完全不同，因此在该器
官中引起的长期感染并非偶然。有关这一点的最惊人数据来自
罗伊·卡尔尼在20世纪60年代的工作，他当时在剑桥大学制订
了肝脏移植计划。《柳叶刀》社论"奇怪的英国猪"中对他的工
作进行了描述，表明了如何突破常规移植障碍来实现没有排异
反应的移植。要了解这一点的重要性，首先必须了解器官移植
中的一个重要问题。

对于其他器官（例如，肾脏、心脏、胰腺和肺），受体的MHC
分子与供体的MHC分子之间必须精确匹配，否则就会产生强 79

烈的免疫反应。尽管乍看之下这可能有些出乎意料，因为接受过训练的宿主T细胞可以识别自身的MHC分子，但事实证明，即使是呈递了无害肽段的外源MHC也会被结合并被识别为病毒。换句话说，外源MHC的总体形状足以与T细胞受体结合并触发免疫反应。这种免疫反应会被进一步加强，因为移植物通过外科手术植入体内，引起组织损伤并通过先天性炎症反应对免疫系统发出了警告。因此，在正常情况下，如果供体和受体的MHC不匹配，那么许多T细胞会聚集到移植物上，这会导致严重的组织损伤，并使移植物被迅速排斥。

　　然而，在肝脏移植中不需要MHC的匹配。此外，成功进行肝脏移植的受体也可以从同一供体那里接受其他器官的移植。换句话说，肝脏移植可使它们对某些外源抗原具有特异的耐受性——移植物并不能使它们具有普遍耐受性，而是只对供体中的MHC分子具有耐受性。在人类的肝脏移植中会发生同样的情况，仅要求供体和受体在血型方面进行匹配，此处的最终接受程度如此之高，以至于在某些情况下不需要使用免疫抑制药物。

　　我们尚不清楚肝脏是如何实现这一点的，但是其中一种机制是通过非常有限的共同刺激来呈递抗原。在这种情况下，检测抗原的T细胞无法有效增殖，并且会提早死亡。肝脏以肝窦内皮细胞的形式包含其专业的抗原呈递细胞群，可以大量摄取和呈递抗原。在没有炎症的情况下，它们可以有效地耐受免疫反应。由于肝脏的血液供应量很大，且细胞在器官内的移动非常缓慢，因此这些相互作用非常频繁且十分有效。

　　肝脏的另一个有趣特征是其内皮有**膜孔**（即，它具有间隙或窗口,可以使血液中的淋巴细胞接触组织细胞,通常情况下,它们必须穿过内皮才能做到这一点)。这一特点意味着,不具备允许其进入组织的归巢受体的幼稚T细胞有可能检测出呈递在该器官上的抗原。免疫反应的有效启动通常发生在淋巴样器官中,并得到其中的树突状细胞、共同刺激分子、细胞因子和基质支撑物等的支持。正如前文所述,在外周组织中首次遇到抗原可能会导致部分激活,因此是无效激活。

为什么会这样设计肝脏?一种说法是,我们需要耐受生活在肠道中的我们自己的微生物以及来自我们所吃食物的抗原。由于来自肠道的所有血液都通过肝脏排出,因此在这种**耐受**环境中呈递抗原是限制反应的一种方法。显然,这需要一种良好的平衡,因为如果通过这种途径进入体内的是一种严重的侵入性病原体,那么肝脏就是在该病原体到达身体其他部位之前阻止其扩散的理想场所,而且肝脏具有一系列限制这种扩散所必需的抵御细菌的能力,尤其是一系列有效的组织驻留巨噬细胞(库普弗细胞),可以吞噬微生物。但是,总的来说,该系统似乎受到了严格的调节或抑制,前文提到的肝炎病毒显然是利用了这种耐受的环境,从而让病毒持久地存在。

另一个需要抑制自然发生的免疫反应的情况是怀孕。胎儿和胎盘均含有来自父亲和母亲的抗原,除非来自父母的抗原存在极为紧密的联系,否则它们其实是不相匹配的移植物,应当发生排异反应。显然,有一套容错机制可以防止这种情况的发生,包括前文提到的机制。实际上,怀孕期间孕妇的整个免疫系统 81 都受到该过程的影响,孕妇的免疫力受到了适度的抑制,因此在此期间孕妇感染某些疾病(例如,水痘带状疱疹和疟疾)的风险较高。

可以限制胎盘中免疫反应的一个有趣因素是免疫代谢的调节。T细胞需要大量的氨基酸才能发挥功能，而其中的一种氨基酸——色氨酸——起着至关重要的作用，因为环境中这种分子的特异性缺失可以阻断T细胞的激活。因此，限制局部环境中的色氨酸是阻止胎盘中免疫反应的有效方法，而这是通过吲哚胺脱氧酶（IDO）来完成的，这种酶可以有效分解色氨酸。IDO并不局限于胎盘，并且确实是在树突状细胞中被激活的，这就允许它们在激活之后调节免疫反应。实验显示，阻断IDO会导致小鼠中胎儿的免疫排异反应，因此表明它在胎儿耐受性中具有重要作用。

肝脏具有自己的可以持续生成的IDO（TDO），并可能有助于在肝脏中提高耐受性。色氨酸不是唯一通过这种方式调节炎症的氨基酸。精氨酸也是必不可少的，精氨酸可以从T细胞中分离出来，并通过精氨酸酶的作用来限制其功能，正如在肿瘤以及一些特殊的与巨噬细胞相关的调节性细胞（被称为髓样抑制细胞）中观察到的那样。

自身免疫性疾病和炎症

在了解了阻止自身免疫的机制，并且了解了如果这些机制失效后会产生的一些严重的综合征之后，让我们来聊一聊一些常见且复杂的自身免疫性疾病和炎症性疾病。其中最广为人知的一种疾病就是类风湿性关节炎（RA），它会导致关节发炎并最终损坏关节，在严重的情况下还会伴有对其他器官造成的炎症性组织损伤。RA的病因尚不清楚，但让我们考虑一个有趣的假设,这个假设汇集了许多已知的线索。

罹患RA的风险高度依赖于特定的MHC分子,尤其是Ⅱ类分子(例如,HLA DRB1*04)。这表明,来自这些分子的特定肽段的呈递是这种疾病的部分原因。显然,这种疾病还与针对特定蛋白质(**瓜氨酸化**蛋白质)的抗体的形成相关。瓜氨酸是精氨酸的一种修饰物,产生于炎症的过程中,并通过改变抗原蛋白的形状为免疫系统创造了一个新的靶点。瓜氨酸肽抗体被用作RA诊断测试的一部分。瓜氨酸肽抗体出现的时间非常早,表明其与发生疾病的原因有关。吸烟与RA的关系也越来越密切,吸烟时间越长,吸烟强度越大,罹患RA的风险就越大。

因此,拉尔斯·克拉雷斯科及其同事提出的一个想法是,吸烟会导致瓜氨酸化蛋白的生成,这些蛋白质可能会形成免疫反应的新靶点。存在危险的HLA分子的情况下,这些新的肽段会被呈递,耐受性会遭到破坏,随后会形成针对这些经过修饰的靶点的抗体。这些自身免疫性反应会影响双侧肺部(即使在临床上并不明显,也会提示RA中的变化)和关节。由于在关节疾病形成很多年之前就已经出现了这种抗体,因此可能需要再次刺激才会引起关节发炎。总而言之,把导致RA的遗传因素和环境因素联系在一起是一个有趣的想法,这也提示了不同类型的RA有不同的病因,因为某些个体并未形成针对瓜氨酸化蛋白质的抗体。RA所涉及的因素如图20所示。

多发性硬化症(MS)是中枢神经系统内发生的由自身免疫性反应导致的潜在破坏性疾病。这种炎症会导致神经周围髓鞘的丢失,从而令其丧失功能。多发性硬化症通常是一种间歇性疾病,发作之后会有一段时间的平静,但随着时间的推移会导致

83

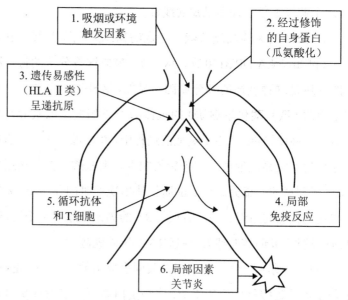

图20 类风湿性关节炎（RA）模型的提出结合了一些已知的遗传诱因和环境诱因。炎症也可能与关节外（例如，肺部或皮肤）疾病症状的形成有关

累积性残疾。像RA一样，多发性硬化症和HLA Ⅱ类基因紧密相关（在这种情况下为DR2复合物，如DRB1*1501），提示了辅助性T细胞在其启动过程中所起的作用。在MS中，遗传因素和环境因素之间也有非常有趣的联系。在北欧和美国等温带气候区（或向这些地区的早期移民中），这种疾病更为普遍；这种疾病在女性中也更为常见，并且与EBV感染的相关程度也越来越高。

EBV感染在全球范围内非常普遍，在某些环境中几乎无所不在，据说有250万人患有MS，因此这不是一个简单的因果关系。一种观点是，来自EBV的肽段和来自脑组织的肽段（例如，髓鞘碱性蛋白）之间存在抗原表位模拟。这种模拟只有当肽段由危险的MHC蛋白质呈递时才会出现，从而解释了其遗传风险。另外，易感染个体大脑中的EBV感染，可以通过提供必要的危险信号（如前文所述）来揭示自身蛋白质的免疫反应并破坏对自身的耐受性。

另一种观点是对疾病的地域性解释，即与缺少光照有关。远离赤道的地区缺少光照，这与较低的维生素D水平有关。这种维生素在免疫系统中具有重要的调节作用，而较低的维生素D水平与自身免疫性疾病有关。有趣的是，影响体内维生素D水平的遗传变异会对罹患MS的风险产生影响，从而加强了这种因果关系。性激素与免疫系统之间存在一些复杂的相互作用，但是较低的睾丸激素水平也可能影响整体的免疫反应，并且还与MS疾病的进展加快有关。

整体而言，脑部炎症的开始和临床疾病的发展之间的一系列步骤正在形成一幅画面。通常情况下，这些步骤可以通过前文描述的所有检查点得到很好的调节，但是一系列的环境风险和遗传风险可能会打破这种平衡，如果不利因素积少成多，就会有利于疾病的发生。幸运的是，正如第七章所述，通过除去其中的某些遗传风险，除了生物制剂将免疫细胞群作为靶点之外，这还为潜在的新疗法敞开了大门（例如，调节维生素D或性激素的水平）。

85

由基因与环境相互作用引起的另一种原因复杂的自身免疫性疾病，是炎症性肠道疾病（IBD）。IBD实际上至少是两种疾病——克罗恩病与肠道深处的裂孔有关，可发生在胃肠道的任何部位（包括口腔及小肠）；而溃疡性结肠炎会导致仅影响大肠的非常严重的炎症。实际上，这两种疾病都可能与肠道外（例如，关节和皮肤）的某些炎症有关，并且这两种疾病本身之间，以及与其他器官的自身免疫性疾病（分别为强直性脊柱炎和银屑病）之间，有着同样的基因风险因素。这表明了炎症的共同通路，并可能是一种重合的病因。

RA和MS会影响通常情况下没有微生物存在的器官（无菌部位），而IBD会影响肠道——肠道是数万亿正常肠道菌落或**微生物群**的家园。许多罕见的遗传缺陷可以导致IBD。IL-10是一种可以有效抑制免疫反应的细胞因子。该分子的丢失或其受体及下游信号的丢失会导致该病的发病非常早。这表明了免疫调节在控制微生物群的反应中的重要作用，而IBD的流行模型就是这种精细的平衡被打破，从而导致持续性的炎症。免疫系统必须在很大程度上忽略肠道中的正常微生物，即使同一种微生物穿过肠道壁几毫米后进入血液就会引起严重的健康威胁。可能存在一个连续的过程，可以非常有效地应对错位的微生物，而无须激活完整的炎症反应；但是，如果真正的病原体试图入侵，这些攻击性反应就很容易发挥作用。

IBD的遗传学特征十分惊人，并指出了导致疾病的两条重要线索。首先是17型防御轴，我们在针对酵母菌的表面防御中遇到过，这是由细胞因子，例如白细胞介素23（IL-23）调节的。影响该轴的基因变异与IBD的风险增加有关。其次，先天免疫反应也很重要，因为这里涉及一个特定的基因NOD2，这是针对细菌的模式识别受体。无法识别和快速处理相对无害的共生细菌，可能会促进肠道内持续进行的免疫反应并形成恶性循环，使肠道受损，从而导致宿主组织进一步暴露于细菌（见图21）。

免疫系统

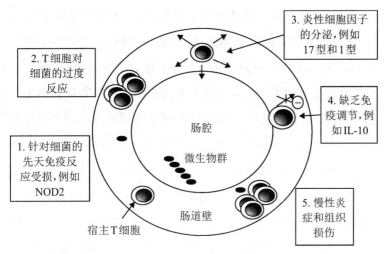

图21　炎症性肠道疾病（IBD）、克罗恩病和溃疡性结肠炎具有很强的遗传易感性,但其发病也需要由环境因素触发（可能是肠道微生物群）

　　有许多有趣的新方法可以抑制此类炎症,例如,细胞因子和趋化因子的特异性阻断（在第七章中有更为详细的讨论）。然而,这种疾病的原因是自身肠道菌群的平衡状态欠佳,这一点对于人类的健康具有更广泛的意义。

　　微生物群非常复杂,只有采用新的分子技术,才有可能从单个个体的肠道中分离出大量的菌群。其中有许多菌群无法通过标准方法进行培养,迄今为止,微生物学家自然而然地专注于与疾病有关的微生物,而忽略了上述微生物。人在出生之后体内就会出现微生物群,随着时间的流逝,宿主和微生物群之间的关系也会不断地进化,每个个体最后都会形成略有不同的平衡状态。该菌群还会通过暴露于PAMPs、细菌抗原以及细菌的代谢产物来调节免疫反应,这对于肠道界面以及整个个体的宿主免疫反应都会产生重要的影响。

最近，这个研究领域吸引了很多关注，不同的微生物群与不同类型的疾病有关，从 IBD、RA、MS 到肥胖、帕金森病和阿尔茨海默病。这种类型的研究仍然处于相对早期的阶段，因此很少能将微生物种群的特定变化与导致疾病的机制紧密联系在一起。然而，如果因果关系得到证实，那么有可能通过调节肠道微生物群来提供一种有趣的附加干预措施，从而预防甚至治疗一系列疾病。应当注意的是，肠道不是身体中唯一具有自身微生物群的部位——即使在肠道内微生物群也会有所变化，而在皮肤和喉咙等不同区域也存在着共生的细菌。这些可能不仅会对局部免疫系统产生影响，而且还可能产生更广泛的影响。

这三个例子都表明了不同的遗传因素和环境因素是如何共同作用从而增加自身免疫性疾病的风险。每个单独的风险可能相对较小，但是所有风险结合在一起就会破坏通过进化形成的抵御自身免疫性疾病的安全防御机制。可用这样的方式来看待这种情况：体内通常存在多个防御层，因此如果自身免疫性反应出现问题，则多个环节都需要出现问题。考虑到每种影响（遗传因素或环境因素）的风险往往很小，因此需要进行大型研究（通常是数千名受影响的患者）来检测其风险。幸运的是，通过遗传技术和**大数据**分析（大量的电子健康数据）已经可以实现上述研究。

过 敏

从某种意义上说，过敏与自身免疫性反应有关，这是免疫系统无法对正常的提示做出响应，从而对不当的抗原做出过度和有害反应的情况。在这种情况下，抗原不是自身性抗原，而是无

88

害（不危险）的非自身性抗原。通过前文提到的耐受性机制，暴露于这类抗原（例如，花粉、室内尘螨的蛋白质、食物）会引起最低程度的反应。然而，对此类抗原的异常反应或超敏反应非常普遍，并且十分危险。

过敏的标志是由一组被称为2型T细胞的特殊T细胞诱导的2型免疫反应（见图22）。2型T细胞倾向于分泌较低水平的抗病毒细胞因子（例如，干扰素γ）并分泌更多不同种类的白细胞介素（尤其是IL-4、IL-5和IL-13），它们能够刺激完全不同的细胞类型和功能。显然，这些细胞并不是为了促进过敏而进化的，其进化的动力似乎是宿主对蠕虫的抵御。蠕虫感染比细菌感染、真菌感染或病毒感染更为复杂，因为入侵的病原体是多细

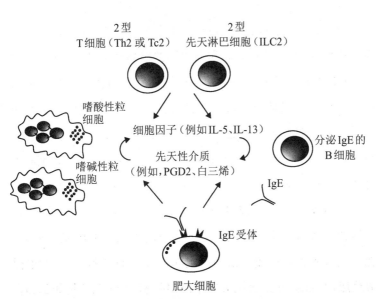

图22　该图展示了2型反应中涉及的一些重要细胞和介质。被2型T细胞和特异性IgE识别的触发性抗原包括无害的蛋白质（例如，来自室内尘螨）、药物和昆虫毒液

胞生物，其体积比抵御它的免疫细胞要大几个数量级，因此不易被吞噬。尽管在现代西方社会中，蠕虫感染很少见，但在人类进化的早期阶段，蠕虫感染是巨大的威胁，目前在世界某些地区仍然如此。因此，针对蠕虫感染的强有力抵御是必不可少的，并需要通过2型反应调动的效应器组合来实现。

在这一过程中被诱导的一组关键细胞是嗜酸性粒细胞。它们来自骨髓，与中性粒细胞有关，但是含有不同的颗粒，因此易于区分。这些颗粒含有特殊的高效分子，可以消化并攻击包括蠕虫在内的组织，其中包括活性氧、蛋白酶和攻击细胞膜的成孔蛋白。它们还会分泌大量介质，从而将更多细胞召集到该部位并激活它们。血液中嗜酸性粒细胞过多是蠕虫感染的标志，也是过敏的标志。

由2型反应引起的过敏反应的另一个重要介质，是一种被称为E类IgE的特殊抗体。和高水平的嗜酸性粒细胞一样，高水平的IgE也和过敏密切相关。在抗原识别端，IgE与任何其他抗体没有区别。但是，该分子的独特之处在于它可以激活存在于特殊的免疫细胞群——肥大细胞——上的一组受体。如果含有激活受体的肥大细胞遇到抗原，例如在皮肤或气道中，则细胞本身就会被迅速激活，从而发出一系列炎症信号。肥大细胞的激活非常高效，因为该细胞中含有预先形成的分子（例如，组胺），可导致组织中的即时炎症反应，这表现为局部的肿胀和刺激。肥大细胞的大量释放通常会产生非常深远的影响，即所谓的**过敏反应**，可能会导致血压突然下降、敏感区域（尤其是面部和舌部）的普遍肿胀、皮疹。这种反应可以通过暴露于IgE已经达到足够水平的任何抗原（包括昆虫叮咬、药物和食物中的蛋白质）

而引起。

过敏反应通常被视为器官特异性疾病，例如，花粉过敏、哮喘或湿疹。通常，这些疾病会发生于单一个体或一个家庭中，并且这种疾病确实有很强的遗传易感性。尽管涉及的许多基因与免疫反应有关，但并非所有基因都是如此。对于湿疹而言，丝聚合蛋白基因的突变会导致皮肤屏障受到细小的破坏，尚不清楚这种情况到底如何导致过敏，但很可能是因为这会暴露于更多的抗原，或者导致免疫系统遇到抗原的情况发生变化，从而提高其意识并促进2型反应。

其他突变会影响2型反应中所涉及的激活不同细胞亚群的相关分子，例如CRTH2。CRTH2是前列腺素D2（肥大细胞释放的重要脂质介质之一）的表面受体。在2型T细胞、嗜酸性粒细胞、嗜碱性粒细胞（相关性密切）以及具有2型偏倚的先天淋巴细胞上均发现了CRTH2。因此，它是2型亚群的独特标志物，也是可阻断前列腺素信号的药物的靶点。前列腺素及其脂类相似物、白三烯都参与了一系列炎症过程，药物孟鲁司特钠对白三烯作用的阻断，长期以来一直被用作治疗哮喘的方法。

尽管一系列细胞都参与了过敏反应，但是只有一些关键通路和信号分子（例如，前列腺素D2或白细胞介素5）是相同的，这与其他免疫环境中遇到的分子截然不同。这种现象为我们提供了一些希望，有望找到针对性更强的哮喘治疗方法。过敏性哮喘是由肺部持续发生的2型反应引起的，这会导致气道发炎和气道收缩。这些特征既互相关联又有所不同。在大多数情况下，目前的治疗都有赖于使用类固醇吸入剂来抑制局部炎症，以及与使用肾上腺素有关的化合物来改善气道收缩。然而，如果病情很严重，则必须口服或静脉内注射大剂量的类固醇以保持气道畅通，但长期使用会引起副作用：骨质疏松、免疫抑制、体重增加。

尽管阻断白细胞介素 5 的生物制剂代表了一种有趣的方法，但仍需要方法来针对性地关闭支持这种严重疾病的 2 型反应。在某些过敏反应中，可能会对免疫反应重新设定程序，并用危害性较小的反应代替 2 型反应。这可以通过脱敏过程来实现，在脱敏过程中会给予皮肤小剂量的抗原，这种剂量不断重复给予并在一段时间内进行积累。我们会观察到，抗原的 IgE 水平（例如，来自蜂毒）下降，而 IgG4 反应可以对其进行取代。IgG4 是一种有趣的分子，几乎不存在激活功能，且可以用作阻断性或抑制性抗体。实际上，这种治疗方法已经存在了一个多世纪，在人们对免疫机制尚未有清晰了解之前，这种治疗方法就已经发展完善，就疫苗而言也是如此。

关于过敏反应，还有许多东西有待学习，例如，为何个体会对一个特定的抗原产生特定的过敏反应，这一点尚不清楚。和自身免疫一样，其中有来自该个体的遗传多态性的成分，以及其所暴露的环境（包括微生物群）。一种流行的理论是**卫生假说**，该理论提出了环境暴露的特定作用。因此，儿童时期暴露于微生物含量较高的环境可以减少发生过敏反应的概率。这个观点具有争议性，但已被提出来用于解释西方社会中过敏性疾病增加的原因。

当然，有数据可以支持上述观点，即儿童所接触的病原体的多样化程度越高（例如，住在农场里会大幅提升病原体的多样性），发生过敏反应的风险就越低。一项针对美国阿米什人和哈特人社区的研究发现,尽管两个群体在许多方面都非常相似,但阿米什儿童的哮喘发病率要低得多。事实证明,阿米什人采用传统的耕作方式,而哈特人采用现代工业化技术,而且阿米什人家中的环境含有广度更大、数量更多的微生物。尚不清楚这种微生物暴露究竟如何通过转移或训练免疫反应来发挥作用,但这是微生物如何对免疫进化产生普遍影响的另一个实例。 93

第六章 免疫力过高:自身免疫性疾病与过敏性疾病

免疫系统 2.0 版：生物疗法和免疫疗法

在前面的章节中，我们讨论了免疫系统的基本组成部分，这些部分如何作为一个整体进行工作，以及如果整体协作未能实现时会发生什么情况。然而，这种基础知识可以应用于对疾病预后的影响，包括免疫学方面的影响和非免疫学方面的影响。在本章中，我们将讨论三个相互联系的主要领域，这些领域可以应用免疫学知识以应对当前的挑战：提高疫苗的免疫力、利用免疫力治疗癌症、研制阻断免疫和自身免疫的新型疗法。我们还将研究与免疫系统老化有关的问题，以及如何纠正这些问题从而治疗或预防疾病。

增强免疫力和疫苗

首先，我们来考虑下如何增强免疫反应，也许最明显的应用形式在疫苗领域。几百年来，疫苗一直对人类健康产生着巨大影响，而研制疫苗的基础免疫学原理也越来越广为人知，但我们仍然缺乏有效的疫苗来治疗一些严重的感染，如HIV、TB和疟疾。为什么会出现这种情况？如何应对这种情况？这三种感染的共同点是具有持久的感染力，这一点与其他复杂疫苗的靶点（例如，HCV、CMV）相同。流感、**流感嗜血杆菌**和麻疹等感染，94往往不会在健康的宿主中引起持续性感染，并且其诱导的免疫力会很强，因此，生成针对流行菌株的高水平抗体的疫苗方法可以提供保护性免疫力。对于流感而言，其面临的挑战在于确定哪些菌株会构成威胁，因为有一些禽流感菌株如果跨物种感染人类，将会非常危险，但所面临的问题仍然相同。对于当前的流感疫苗而言，提供当季流行的相关病毒类型的蛋白质（使用在鸡蛋上培育的病毒），再辅以佐剂，就可以增强先天免疫反应，这通常足以诱导中和抗体达到保护性水平。而麻疹的疫苗是天然病毒的减毒活疫苗，可以提供终身的免疫力。

然而，正如我们在HIV感染中看到的一样，生成针对病毒包膜的抗体可以中和某些菌株，但是很容易被其他菌株逃避，因此只能提供有限的保护。一项目的在于诱导HIV包膜抗体的试验（RV144，泰国）显示，其在预防感染方面取得了部分成功，并让人产生了能够研制出有效抗体的希望，但要使用这种抗体还有很长的路要走，因为这种抗体的保护水平仅有30%。进一步优化所使用的抗原，并将抗体反应集中于可以中和多种变体的领域，可能会增强这种疫苗的保护水平。

有望通过其他方式来利用T细胞反应从而提供保护。这将依靠CD8+ T细胞清除受感染细胞中的感染情况，因此这与前文中提到的疫苗使用方法完全不同。人们已经尝试过这种方法，但是并没有成功，而且有人担心疫苗甚至可能会增加HIV携带者的感染风险。可能T细胞需要靶向定位病毒中正确的肽段。95

来自路易斯·皮克尔实验室的一种方法是，利用CMV作为载体（携带病毒）来呈递HIV蛋白。这些实验中使用的CMV可能会破坏MHC Ⅰ类呈递的某些方面，这显然是在迫使免疫系统使用其他呈递分子，这种情况下人体使用的分子是HLA-E。

HLA-E不具有多态性，通常会向NK细胞呈递一组有限的肽段；但就目前仅用于猴子的这种疫苗而言，它可以呈递病毒的肽段。针对这些肽段的免疫反应非常强烈，与正常的免疫反应完全不同，它们在抑制感染方面非常有效。这些实验提供了一些理论证据，即如果能安全地转化为人体研究，就可以证明基于T细胞的方法具有可行性。

病毒载体疫苗，即利用另一种病毒将目标病原体呈递给免疫系统的疫苗（见图23），确实拥有巨大的潜力。可以设计能将靶点抗原（例如，来自TB、寨卡病毒或埃博拉病毒的抗原）呈递给免疫系统的安全病毒，而其中一些病毒（例如，腺病毒）能够引发极强的免疫反应。这意味着没有必要在实验室中培育病原体，而且理论上免疫反应可以专门针对目标区域进行。也可以把DNA本身作为一种疫苗，注入的DNA将被细胞用于产生目标蛋白质，疫苗可能会引发足够的先天免疫反应来启动新的T细胞和B细胞。DNA疫苗在小鼠中非常有效，但在人体内的效果却相对较差。实际上，这一领域的障碍之一就是，许多在实验室中十分有效的疫苗方法却无法在人类志愿者身上诱导出强烈的免疫反应。

因此，在研制针对复杂病原体的疫苗中，一些困难在于无法了解哪种免疫反应具有保护性，以及无法确定要攻击的靶点；另一些困难则是由于无法利用当前的方法诱导免疫反应。在这两

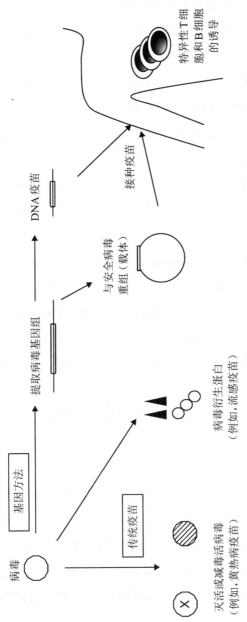

图23 传统疫苗使用减毒株、灭活微生物或病原体衍生的蛋白质。对于更为复杂或危险的病原体，基因方法可以提供替代的疫苗策略

种困难中，后一种困难更容易解决，因为随着对先天免疫反应以及抗原呈递的了解日益加深，再加上用来呈递抗原的分子工具的多样化程度越来越高，这个问题就可以得到解决。确定保护性免疫反应并且试图精确地复制这种反应则要困难得多，即使使用模拟人类疾病的动物模型也是如此，因此，在某些情况下可能仍需反复试验。目前缺乏有效疫苗策略的两种特别复杂的疾病是疟疾和TB。这两种疾病与HIV有一些共同的特征：疟疾的变异性非常高，这使得宿主的反应很难跟上病原体的变异；而TB则拥有一个很难清除的潜藏的感染抗原库，意味着可能存在再次感染的持续威胁。

实际上，随着时间的推移，通过持续暴露于抗原可以产生对疟疾的免疫力。虽然儿童和婴儿感染疟疾十分危险，会产生非常严重的疾病，但是在疟疾流行地区（例如，撒哈拉以南非洲地区）的成年人感染疟疾后受到的影响很小，甚至不会出现临床影响。我们在确定限制此类个体感染的机制方面已经花费了很多精力（有趣的是，如果这些个体离开疾病流行地区，就会丧失这种有效的免疫力），并研制出一种疫苗——RTS, S。然而，这种使用HBV将疟疾抗原呈递给免疫系统的疫苗仅对部分婴儿有效，而且疫苗的效果会随着时间不断减弱，因此这中间还有许多工作有待完成。疟原虫具有复杂的生活方式，其中包括在蚊虫叮咬后穿过肝脏但还未进入红细胞之前的关键阶段。如果可以阻断肝脏中的感染，就可以产生非常有效的免疫力。使用病毒载体疫苗，或者甚至使用经过辐射的整个疟原虫，从而将抗疟疾的T细胞反应导入肝脏的方法，可以产生十分有效的免疫力（见图24）。

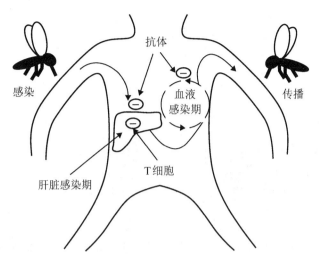

图24 疟原虫通过蚊虫叮咬进行传播,必须进入肝脏才能引起感染。通过疫苗和自然暴露诱导的抗体和T细胞可在不同节点阻断该过程

　　TB由Mtb引起(请参见第二章),主要通过感染者排痰性咳嗽产生的气溶胶飞沫进行传播。世界上约三分之一人口的体内都含有这种微生物,该微生物生命周期中的关键步骤是,能够在其感染的主要细胞——巨噬细胞——中形成长时间的潜伏期。该细菌能够控制巨噬细胞的细胞内环境来提高其存活率,并逃避免疫清除。由于该细菌位于细胞内,关键的免疫反应将由T细胞介导,而T细胞免疫功能的缺陷会导致TB的重新激活。T细胞会分泌干扰素γ和TNFα等细胞因子,它们可以激活巨噬细胞并增强清除作用。T细胞和巨噬细胞之间的这种相互影响会导致**肉芽肿**的形成;肉芽肿是一个复杂的免疫细胞团,其中心部位含有引起免疫反应的细菌(见图25)。

　　针对TB的T细胞疫苗已经以BCG的形式存在了将近一个世纪,BCG是由巴黎巴斯德研究所研制的。这种疫苗——一种

99

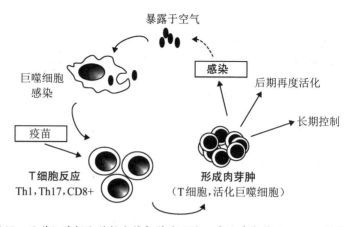

暴露于空气

感染

巨噬细胞
感染

后期再度活化

长期控制

疫苗

T细胞反应
Th1, Th17, CD8+

形成肉芽肿
（T细胞，活化巨噬细胞）

图25　巨噬细胞摄取结核分枝杆菌（Mtb）。在大多数情况下，Mtb持续存在于肉芽肿中并在后期可以再度活化。如果T细胞的免疫反应较弱，则Mtb可能会在肺部进一步扩散

在培育过程中形成的TB的减毒株——确实可以生成针对Mtb抗原的高水平T细胞反应。这种疫苗在预防婴儿疾病方面非常有效，而婴儿一旦感染了Mtb就会出现非常严重的情况，病毒会扩散到全身甚至大脑（即，脑膜炎）。然而，BCG对成人的疗效要差得多，且至今尚未研制出新的疫苗。这种现象的原因尚不清楚，但有一个问题是，我们不知道实现保护的关键介质是什么，因此也不知道疫苗的靶点是什么。一旦我们确定了明确的靶点，加上诱导人体内T细胞免疫反应的方法如今已经十分先进，那么新的TB疫苗策略就可以为这一重大的全球性健康问题提供突破性的预防方法。

　　研发新疫苗显然十分重要。首先就是要研发针对RSV（请参见第四章）的疫苗，RSV是一种无处不在的病毒，我们所有人都暴露其中，并且会在婴幼儿中引起严重的疾病。针对RSV的疫苗将在全球范围内带来巨大的益处，但是20世纪60年代尝试

100

生产的针对RSV的疫苗与接种者的疾病发生率和死亡率增加有关。这很可能是由于针对该疫苗——这种疫苗是经过福尔马林处理过的灭活病毒——所形成的异常2型免疫反应所致。因此，增强的免疫反应是非保护性的，反而会导致针对病毒的超敏反应，并使肺部炎症加重。

尽管如此，我们仍在继续尝试研制针对RSV的疫苗，利用我们对免疫系统的不断了解来避免这个危险的问题：或是通过使用病毒载体来呈递RSV抗原，或是为母亲接种疫苗让母体把增强的IgG抗体传给婴儿，从而为婴儿提供被动保护。婴儿体内的保护性抗体的水平会随着时间而下降，但这也意味着在婴儿最脆弱的阶段可以避免感染。越来越多的证据表明，当免疫反应减弱时（将在本章的后文中进行讨论），RSV也会在老年人中引起疾病，这时疫苗可以增强针对RSV的抗体和T细胞反应，从而预防该年龄段的人群受到严重感染。

总体而言，针对常见疾病的疫苗已经挽救了无数生命，并将继续挽救更多的生命——疫苗不仅可以保护接种了疫苗的个体，还可以提供群体免疫，从而限制严重感染的传播。在近期关于使用特定疫苗的争议中，群体免疫的问题已经成为人们关注的焦点。由于疫苗的接种对象是健康的人，因此必须权衡接受保护所带来的好处，以及可能产生的不利因素的风险。幸运的是，由于其中一些感染的影响十分巨大，而疫苗带来的风险又非常小，因此对疫苗的权衡结果倾向于有利的一侧。如果使用针对主要病原体（例如，本章中提到的那些病原体）的下一代疫苗可以达到相同的平衡和结果，则有可能对数百万生命产生积极的影响。

利用免疫反应和癌症的免疫疗法

增强免疫力不仅与感染有关,而且与癌症有关(见图26)。过去十年中,最激动人心的突破之一就是研发利用抗癌免疫反应以使患者受益的新技术。来自HIV(和其他免疫抑制状态)的证据已经表明,免疫反应在控制癌症——主要是由病毒引起的癌症——中起着重要作用。然而,大多数癌症不含作为潜在靶点的病毒蛋白,而只是自身的突变形式。考虑到我们在上一章中讨论过的多层耐受性,这会让针对自身的免疫反应大幅减弱;此外,癌症会表现出某种类似感染的症状,经历选择以避免被淘汰。

因此,研发针对癌症的有效细胞免疫反应被认为是一项非常困难的任务。另一方面,在这个领域人们也不时地取得了一

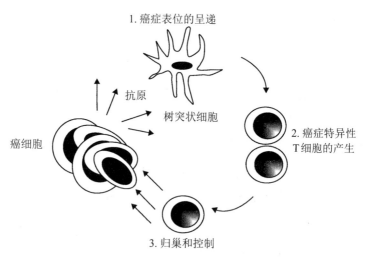

图26 癌症的某些特征会限制针对癌症的特异性免疫反应。这些消极的影响不仅会作用于免疫反应的诱导阶段(树突状细胞),也会作用于效应阶段(在肿瘤微环境中)

些成功：一些患者对疫苗接种或特异性T细胞的转移表现出显著的反应性，这使得人们对这种方法保持持续乐观的态度。在观察癌症的结果并研究肿瘤中的细胞和基因时，有迹象表明，肿瘤中的免疫反应越强，患者的生存状况越好。用于检验数千名患有三十种不同类型癌症的患者预后情况的最新数据显示，肿瘤中与良好预后密切相关的单个基因是免疫基因KLRB1，用于编码CD161——一种在T细胞和NK细胞亚群上表达的具有增强功能的分子。

这种T细胞在癌症中可以识别出什么？一种答案是对癌症本身进行分析，这是宿主细胞DNA遗传突变的结果。每次出现一个重要的突变时，就会形成一个不存在于胸腺中且耐受性从未受到诱导的新的肽段靶点。如果这种肽段可以与患者的MHC分子结合并呈递给T细胞，那么它就是一种**新表位**，即一种识别和杀死肿瘤细胞的合适靶点。有趣的是，某些突变过程加速的肿瘤（由于失去了对细胞复制机制的校对作用）实际上得到了更好的控制，并伴随着更强烈的免疫反应，可能是靶向针对大量生成的新表位。新的癌症基因组测序方法的出现，有可能鉴定出单个癌症患者中出现的新表位。从原理上讲，用疫苗方法靶向针对新表位可能会形成定制的癌症疗法。

然而，T细胞反应还须克服组织中存在的耐受性效应，尤其是抑制分子提供的检查点。近期，用单克隆抗体阻断这种检查点的能力，对这一领域产生了最重大的影响。对PD-1和CTLA4 等抑制性分子的阻断，可以对癌症的控制产生巨大影响，结合使用（而无需其他治疗方法）可显著延长晚期黑色素瘤（最具侵袭性的癌症之一）患者的无病生存期。黑色素瘤是一种有趣的肿

103

瘤,因为它们含有免疫系统的既定靶点,并在过去对免疫疗法有所反应。目前,阻断检查点这一方法已被应用于一系列其他类型的肿瘤中,例如肺癌和肾癌。正如人们所预期的那样,其缺点是会诱导自身免疫现象(肠道炎症尤为常见),但是考虑到这对于癌症本身的预后来说,如果控制得当,这些自身免疫现象在很大程度上是可以接受的。

有多种机制可以调节健康组织和肿瘤中的T细胞功能,因此人们希望这一成功能为将来进行抗肿瘤反应提供一系列选择,但这种方法确实取决于潜在活跃的T细胞反应的存在。因此,它也可能通过与疫苗接种(如本章所述)或淋巴细胞注射法(即所谓的细胞疗法)一起来增强抗肿瘤反应。

细胞疗法的一种新型方式是形成所谓的嵌合抗原受体T(CAR-T)细胞,经过专门设计的TCR可以针对癌症患者做出反应。这可以让新的T细胞靶向针对癌细胞,T细胞会被激活并形成效应器功能。通过在TCR上构建抗体结构域,可以非常精确地实现这种靶向,因此,这不依赖于经过加工的肽段的呈递,而是依赖于癌症抗原在细胞表面的表达。与此类靶点结合的抗体的特异性非常高且非常有效。这种方法也很有趣,因为T细胞可以一直处于循环状态,并提供长期保护以防止复发。人们正在使用经过专门设计的可溶性TCR来研发类似的方法,选择这些可溶性TCR的原因在于,它们可以非常牢固地与肿瘤靶点结合(由于在胸腺中其强力黏合性被消除,因此在通常情况下TCR相对较弱)。这些能够通过设计实现:当上述TCR与其靶点结合时,就可以召集效应性T细胞并直接在肿瘤部位激活这些T细胞,从而极大地增加了参与抗肿瘤反应的细胞数量。

阻断免疫力和生物疗法

一方面，我们对耐受性机制的理解，可以使我们在出现癌症反应的情况下阻断这种机制并加强炎症；另一方面，对炎症基本机制的了解可以提示阻断自身免疫性反应的策略。实现这种阻断的最有趣的新方法，取决于对免疫反应本身的适应，从而形成基于单克隆抗体的**生物疗法**，这是由塞萨尔·米尔斯坦和乔治斯·克勒共同发明的，他们与尼尔斯·杰尼共同获得了当年的诺贝尔奖。

单克隆抗体来自正常的抗体反应，该抗体甚至对同一抗原也包含许多不同形式的抗体反应。为了得到单克隆抗体的单一、纯化的形式，克勒和米尔斯坦将B细胞**与永生的**癌细胞（即在实验室条件下可以持续分裂并无限生长的细胞）融合在一起，从而形成一系列**杂交瘤**。这些永生的细胞都会分泌一种抗体，不过每个细胞生成的抗体都具有独特的设计结构。通过大规模地进行此项操作，然后筛选所得的杂交瘤，使其与所选的抗原（在最初的研究中是绵羊红细胞，但可以是引起抗体反应的任何物质）进行结合，就有可能得到那些具有正确特异性的杂交瘤。由于杂交瘤是永生的，这使得免疫学家可以制造出几乎无限量的针对已选靶点的高纯度和特异性抗体。尽管已经研制出更新型、更灵活的替代技术，但人们仍在使用这项技术。

单克隆抗体可精确阻断免疫系统的特定方面或靶向针对病原体。尽管20世纪70年代米尔斯坦和克勒已经发明了这些工具，但人们经过一段时间才意识到这些工具的治疗潜力。这项研究首先研制的是针对肿瘤坏死因子α（TNFα）的单克隆抗体。

肿瘤坏死因子α具有高度促炎性,参与多种不同的自身免疫性反应和炎症性反应,并在宿主防御中起着关键作用。TNFα的单克隆抗体疗法的最初应用场景是脓毒症——一种死亡率很高的严重血液感染疾病。正如许多针对这种情况的治疗方法一样,它并没有获得成功。然而,马克·费尔德曼和拉文德·梅尼曾一直致力于对RA中TNFα的研究,并在实验室中研究出了这种方法的阻断作用,而在一项针对这种无效条件下的患者的小型实验中,他们可以重新利用这种被称为**英夫利昔单抗**的治疗方法。这项实验的时间是1992年,实验效果相当显著,很大一部分患者都受益于单克隆抗体,并在随后的几十年中为大量这类生物治疗方法的研究铺平了道路。TNFα阻断剂(使用英夫利昔单抗和其他生物学疗法)现已用于多种炎症的治疗,包括IBD(克罗恩病和溃疡性结肠炎)、强直性脊柱炎和银屑病性关节炎。

　　生物疗法可以精确阻断与炎症有关的特定通路,从而避免使用广谱免疫抑制疗法,如类固醇。然而,从这些分子在宿主防御中的作用就可以预测其副作用。TNFα对TB的控制十分重要,即使在其他免疫防御机制完好的情况下,使用这种药物治疗的患者仍有重新感染的风险。此外,尽管该分子已经被设计成"人源化"分子(最初是在小鼠中研制的),但在某些患者中,它仍然可以引起抗体反应,从而限制其有效性。并非所有罹患RA(或提及的其他疾病)的患者都会对此类药物产生反应。这表明,尽管RA看起来是一种疾病,但它在不同患者中起作用的根本机制可能并不相同,因此需要对这些昂贵且具有潜在危险性的治疗方法做进一步的患者分层,这也是现代医学中的一个共同主题。

106

除了TNFα之外，单克隆抗体还可以靶向针对许多其他的细胞因子通路。前文中提到的17型通路，是导致炎症性疾病以及防止细菌和酵母菌感染的一个原因。IL-23是一种促进这种反应的细胞因子，对IL-23的阻断在关节和肠道的炎症性反应中也非常有效。有趣的是，对IL-17本身的阻断可以有效治疗强直性脊柱炎（一种脊椎的发炎性疾病）和银屑病，这些疾病彼此之间以及与IBD之间都具有许多共同的遗传风险因素。然而，阻断IBD中的IL-17实际上会使炎症恶化，其可能原因是宿主对细菌的反应降低，从而加剧了原始的损伤。因此，从某种意义上讲，这些临床研究本身就是实验，一旦一条通路被阻断就会揭示潜在疾病的其他方面，或是揭示特定通路在宿主防御中的作用。

靶向和特异性阻断慢性炎症患者的炎症性通路的能力，对科学家和公司都极具吸引力，目前有许多正在试验中或者已经可以使用的此类产品。阻断其他炎症性细胞因子或其受体（例如，白细胞介素1b和白细胞介素6）的单克隆抗体也可以用于关节炎的治疗，对于那些对TNFα阻断没有反应的人来说，这可能是另外的选择。阻断IL-5和潜在的IL-13则是对过敏和哮喘的干预。这些药物具有足够的潜力来影响这些炎症性疾病，不过研发此类药物的成本非常高，因此在选择正确的靶点时必须格外谨慎。

107

其他基于单克隆抗体疗法的方法包括细胞耗竭——实际上，通过其表面受体CD52靶向针对T细胞的坎帕斯1，是由剑桥大学的赫尔曼·瓦尔德曼研发的首批此类疗法之一。现在被称为阿伦单抗的这种消耗性抗体，可以对MS的病程产生实质性影响，并且是针对这种疾病真正有效的少数疗法之一。使用单克隆抗体的细胞耗竭方法也可以有效治疗癌症。阿伦单抗可用于特定的淋巴瘤，从而破坏正在增殖的淋巴细胞，但更重要的是，利妥昔单抗靶向针对B细胞上的CD20分子，是治疗多种淋巴瘤的有效方法。通过耗竭B细胞（其中多数B细胞表达CD20分子，并且是该药物的靶点），利妥昔单抗还可以重置免疫系统，并用于关闭RA以及一系列自身免疫条件下的抗体反应。就像前文提到的英夫利昔单抗一样，关于这些分子的故事包含了丰富的信息。尽管这些药物是针对单一条件或应用而引入的，但它们可以在多种情况下进行使用，包括在不太可能研发特定药物的相对罕见的情况下或"孤儿"条件下进行使用。

单克隆抗体和生物疗法也可以用于阻断细胞向特定组织的迁移。维多珠单抗是一种特异性整合素的阻断剂，可以让细胞归巢于肠道这一IBD的治疗活跃区。那他珠单抗是一个相关的分子，对淋巴细胞向肠道和大脑的归巢作用会产生影响，可用于治疗MS。然而，未能使得淋巴细胞对大脑组织进行检查这一情况并非不存在风险，因为可能发生由JC病毒引起的严重病毒感染的罕见病例。这种情况也出现于晚期HIV患者中，与严重的免疫抑制有关，且预后极差。在其他情况下也确实会出现这种病毒的再激活现象，尽管有些情况是可预见且可预防的（例如，慢性HBV的再激活），但还有许多情况无法预见且无法预防，因此即使使用这种靶向治疗，也必须格外谨慎（见图27）。

治疗炎症性疾病需要关闭免疫反应，移植也需要关闭免疫反应，在这种情况下单克隆抗体也起着作用。此外，我们已经尝试利用多种技术来诱导耐受性。基于细胞疗法的一个有趣想法是转移调节性T细胞。表达高水平IL-2受体CD25并标记调节

108

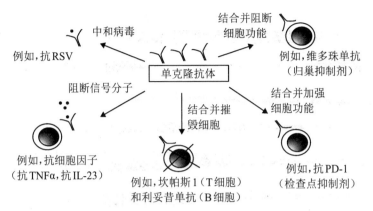

图27 单克隆抗体可精确阻断免疫系统的特定方面或靶向针对病原体。其结合细胞并杀死细胞的能力可用于免疫疗法和癌症治疗

细胞的 CD4+ T 细胞，可以从外周血液中分离出来，在实验室条件下进行培养，然后输送给受体。也可以在体外处理这些细胞以增强其抑制能力。在临床前研究中，这种方法非常有效；尽管有许多实际的障碍需要克服，但人们仍有很大的热情让其为人类所用。调节细胞疗法在自身免疫性疾病中也可能起到作用，并具有潜在的优势，可以相对特异性地减弱异常免疫反应，而不会造成严重的感染。

炎症和衰老（"炎症性衰老"）

最后，让我们来展望未来。我们当前面临的一个问题是老年病的问题，在这些疾病中免疫反应可能需要上调或下调（见图28）。阿尔茨海默病并非像 RA 或 MS 那样被认为是一种自身免疫性疾病，但是通过对受影响人群的研究以及对大量人群的遗传分析可知，越来越多的证据表明免疫反应与阿尔茨海默病有关。TREM2 是一种与阿尔茨海默病有关的基因，该基因

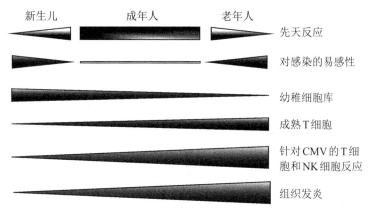

新生儿	成年人	老年人	
			先天反应
			对感染的易感性
			幼稚细胞库
			成熟T细胞
			针对CMV的T细胞和NK细胞反应
			组织发炎

图28　衰老与许多免疫变化有关,这些变化会影响对感染的易感性和对炎症的调节。CMV感染会导致非常强烈的免疫反应,并与这些影响有关

似乎会影响大脑中与巨噬细胞相关的小胶质细胞的功能。目前尚不清楚TREM2究竟如何影响痴呆过程的发展或进展,但它提供了一个潜在的新的治疗机会,来干预这种毁灭性的流行疾病。

　　炎症可能会加速衰老,即所谓的"炎症性衰老"。这是一个非常复杂的领域,因为其中涉及众多因素,而且要区分健康性衰老和早衰并不容易。可能起到作用的一个因素是由感染引起的慢性炎症。许多研究都表明罪魁祸首是CMV,一种世界上多数人口都携带的病毒,其休眠及重新激活的能力意味着需要持续的免疫监视。由于参与这项工作的淋巴细胞数量很多,并且与免疫系统的早衰和反应性的丢失有关,这就导致了免疫系统的明显偏倚性。越来越多的数据表明,在部分个体中,失去对CMV的控制会导致病毒的再度激活和炎症的发生。由于病毒能够在血管壁(内皮细胞)中存活,因此可能导致血管性疾病。需要进一步的大型研究来证实这一特定的假设,如

110

果能证明这一假设为真，那么就能为终止衰老过程提供一个有趣的机会。

此外，研究针对老龄人口的疫苗策略和维持有效免疫反应的其他干预措施，在未来将会变得越来越重要。最近的一项研究想法专注于免疫细胞的代谢，特别是一种被称为**自噬**或自我吞食的过程。自噬是一种对细胞内容物进行循环利用以维持细胞存活的机制，自噬过程由饥饿触发。已有大量数据表明，刺激自噬的过程可以延长寿命。对于淋巴细胞而言，需要自噬的过程来维持长期记忆。在一项实验中，通过使用一种被称为亚精胺的分子，来触发T细胞记忆明显受损的老年小鼠的自噬过程，就会让其记忆T细胞的反应得到明显的改善。这表明免疫衰老过程至少具有部分可逆性，并且简单的干预措施（例如，食物中的亚精胺）有助于这一恢复过程。自噬也可以由许多其他方式引起，包括限制卡路里摄入和运动。因此，有许多方法都可能影响这一关键通路并增强衰老的免疫系统。可能还存在其他的通路会随着年龄的增长而限制免疫力或免疫调节，但目前对于这些通路研究较少。

有趣的是，自噬受到饮食和运动的高度调节。营养状况对这种基本细胞过程的整体影响可能非常重要，免疫系统代谢调节的作用也具有重要意义。例如，维生素和矿物质等微量营养素可以调节T细胞的效应器和调节功能。糖尿病是西方老龄人口中一个日益严重的问题，糖尿病与免疫功能下降以及对感染的易感性增加有关。需要做进一步的机制及临床研究来更好地确定，饮食和生活方式中特定的干预措施，是否会影响所有年龄段人群中的免疫反应和炎症过程。

免疫系统的未来

在本书中,我们探讨了免疫反应的基本构成要素(人类通过进化继承了这些要素),以及免疫系统如何协调自身的功能来平衡攻击性(对抗危险病原体)和耐受性(自身及微生物群)。通常情况下,免疫系统的工作完成得十分出色,以至于我们忽视了其对于日常生活的影响,只有在免疫系统出现故障时我们才会注意到它的存在。在第一章中,我们讨论了免疫系统如何对全身产生影响,以及我们如何日渐意识到炎症过程涉及从癌症到痴呆症的许多疾病。

进化可能会调整我们的免疫系统,让我们熬过生命中的前几十年,因此本章前文中讨论的问题可能是这种早期偏倚的结果。在全球范围内,我们面临许多传染性疾病,如HIV、疟疾和TB。预防和治疗这些疾病将取决于对免疫系统的靶点的进一步理解,以及找到更具可行性的系统来诱导保护性T细胞和B细胞的免疫反应。这是自疫苗接种领域的先驱人物詹纳和巴斯德以来一直在进行的延伸性工作,由于对基础免疫学和微生物学的认识不断加深,对预防和治疗方法改进的程度也在不断提升。通过研发疫苗来利用免疫系统,已经获得了巨大的成功。

在21世纪,尤其是在发达国家,人们面临的主要疾病是心血管疾病和癌症,但随着人口结构的不断变化,痴呆症和老年病的比重也在不断上升。对于免疫学家而言,这是一个全然不同的挑战,但是由于免疫系统涉及整个人体和许多重要的病理过程,因此这是一个必须要面对的挑战。使用基于单克隆抗体技术的小分子药物或生物分子对炎症性通路进行特异性阻断,

112

为我们提供了在新环境中调节免疫反应的一套重要工具。鉴于这些方法在典型的自身免疫性疾病和炎症性疾病（例如，RA和IBD）方面取得的巨大进步，因此我们可以乐观地应对新的挑战。对老龄人口的免疫系统进行调整或重新训练，从而令其有效地运转——增强抵抗感染的能力，同时预防慢性炎症——对于该领域的研究者来说是一项过于复杂而无法独立应对的任务，因此需要许多来自其他领域的支持。然而，随着我们对与这些疾病有关的免疫通路的剖析，这将为我们个人和全社会在面临上述疾病和其他疾病的情况下，继续提供新的治疗机会和预防措施。

索 引

(条目后的数字为原文页码,
见本书边码)

113

索
引

115

Paul Klenerman

THE IMMUNE SYSTEM

A Very Short Introduction

Contents

Acknowledgements

I would like thank all the people who have helped me prepare this book. First, my colleagues at the Peter Medawar Building and Translational Gastroenterology Unit at Oxford, who have looked at various drafts, including Nick Provine, Philippa Matthews, Susie Dunachie, and Matt Bilton. Also to Chris Willberg and Alba Llibre who provided the pictures of germinal centres and to Philip Goulder, my longstanding office-mate, who put up with me and kept my plants alive. Huge thanks must go to David Greaves from the Dunn School of Pathology at Oxford, who spent many hours of his time helping and educating me, especially about macrophages. I am very grateful to my past teachers in immunology, Herman Waldmann and Alan Munro at Cambridge, Andrew McMichael and Rodney Phillips at Oxford, Hans Hengartner and Rolf Zinkernagel (and his viruses) in Zurich, who brought the subject to life for me and one way or another have all contributed to the ideas in the book. Thanks must go to those who have funded me and my lab, especially the Wellcome Trust, who have supported my work through their fellowship scheme from the start. I have also had excellent support from the National Institutes of Health Research (which funds Oxford's Biomedical Research Centre), the Oxford Martin School, Medical Research Council, National Institutes for Health (USA), and Cancer Research UK for different projects in infection and immunity. Finally I must thank my family hugely—my wife Sally and children Tom and Emma—for all the love, enthusiasm, and energy they bring, and for making me explain stuff properly. I would like to dedicate the book to my parents, Leslie and Naomi Klenerman (respectively, the author of and the spark behind *Human Anatomy: A Very Short Introduction*), who encouraged me to write this in the first place, but who did not live to see it completed. Their memory (immunological and otherwise) lives on.

List of illustrations

The Immune System

List of abbreviations

AID	activation-induced cytosine deaminase
AIDS	Acquired Immunodeficiency Syndrome
BCG	Bacille Calmette–Guérin
bNABs	broadly neutralizing antibodies
CAR-T	chimeric antigen receptor
CF	cystic fibrosis
CMV	cytomegalovirus
CRISPR	clustered, regularly interspaced, short palindromic repeats
CRP	C reactive protein
CVID	common variable immunodeficiency
DAMPs	damage-associated molecular patterns
EBV	Epstein–Barr Virus
HBV	Hepatitis B Virus
HCV	Hepatitis C Virus
HIV	Human Immunodeficiency Virus
HLA	Human Leukocyte Antigen
HMBPP	4-Hydroxy-3-methyl-but-2-enyl pyrophosphate
HPV	Human Papilloma Virus
IBD	inflammatory bowel disease
IDO	indoleamine deoxygenase
ILCs	innate lymphoid cells
LCMV	Lymphocytic Choriomeningitis Virus
LPS	lipopolysaccharide
MAIT	mucosal-associated invariant T
MHC	Major Histocompatibility Complex
Mtb	*Mycobacterium tuberculosis*
MS	multiple sclerosis

NET	neutrophil extracellular trap
NK	natural killer
NOD2	nucleotide-binding oligomerization domain-containing protein 2
PAMPs	pathogen-associated molecular patterns
PD-1	programmed death 1
RA	rheumatoid arthritis
RAG	recombination activating gene
RSV	Respiratory Syncitial Virus
siRNA	short-interfering RNA
SIVs	Simian Immunodeficiency Viruses
TB	tuberculosis
TCR	T cell receptor
TGFb	Tissue Growth Factor beta
TLR	Toll-like receptor
TNFa	Tumor Necrosis Factor alpha

The Immune System

Chapter 1
What is the immune system?

The immune system and immunity

The concept of immunity is familiar to most of us. The idea
of remaining healthy in the face of an infectious disease is a
powerful one, and is akin to being exempt from some unpleasant
duty or tax. The word 'immunity' derives from the Latin meaning
'uncommon' or 'privileged'. The idea might have emerged from the
observation that the average person would be susceptible to the
disease, and the unusual one would be protected or immune.

Although this idea of immunity is very clearly understood in the
context, say, of an epidemic—a situation where most individuals
may be infected with only a few being immune—it hides a perhaps
less recognized feature. We now understand that the immune
system is keeping us healthy continuously—the basic elements
of the immune system are so effective that it is only when it is
defective that we become susceptible to specific types of disease.
In other words, through evolution, the function of the immune
system has been honed so that many infectious organisms are dealt
with very effectively, either eliminated from the body or held at bay
without the individual succumbing to any significant illness.

New *pathogens* (micro-organisms that can cause disease),
especially those that cross over from other species to infect

humans (such as Ebola), can create a series of new challenges to the immune system—but fortunately it is designed to rise above even such previously unseen threats. However, there are many other organisms which only cause disease when immune structures or defence systems are damaged or underdeveloped, such as in the neonate, or through a mutation in a specific gene. Such infections—for example, those caused by certain types of bacteria and yeasts—are often termed *opportunistic* (i.e. they only lead to disease under certain conditions). One famous example is that of 'the boy in the bubble', David Vetter, whose immune system was so deficient that even simple bodily contact put him at risk of severe infection. It is examples such as these—'experiments of nature' or mutations which can be studied in laboratory conditions—that have taught us an enormous amount about the normal function of the immune system in what might be termed 'everyday' host defence. In the words of Joni Mitchell—if out of context—'you don't know what you've got till it's gone'.

The immune system resists not only threats from the outside but also those emerging from within. The immune system can be regarded as a system to maintain the status quo within the body—so-called *homeostasis*. Thus in the presence of an organism invading from the outside, the immune system is activated to eliminate it. However, when, say, abnormal tissue changes occur within an individual in the form of cancer (transformation of normally regulated tissue to abnormal tissue which has escaped from natural controls over growth and localization), here the immune system also has a role to play, and this is increasingly being recognized. In some (fortunately rare) cases, the cancer may in fact be driven by a micro-organism—for example, viruses are involved in the development of cervical cancer (Human Papilloma Virus or HPV) and some lymphatic cancers (lymphomas, caused for example by Epstein Barr Virus). Here the immune system is potentially able to respond to the virus causing the cancer. In many other settings, it is potentially able to recognize the changes within the cancer tissue itself. There are many checks and balances on this recognition as we will discuss later in the book, but one of the most exciting features of modern immunology is the realization that immune responses can be harnessed to provide new effective treatments for cancers.

One other important feature of immune systems is drawn out by the nature of the micro-organisms they are designed to resist. Bacteria and viruses have relatively small *genomes* (the total amount of genetic information in an organism) compared to their hosts—some viruses such as parvoviruses only encode for two full genes compared to our complement of around 20,000. Viruses can be based on RNA or DNA genomes—they can both hold the same types of genetic information but simply represent different viral lifestyles. They replicate these genomes fast and on a massive scale (there may be many millions of copies of viruses in every millilitre of blood during a viral infection). This allows the process of mutation and natural selection to work very quickly. In some cases, this is even accentuated by the copying mechanisms used—certain RNA-based viruses have *polymerases* (proteins which copy the genome and thus replicate the virus) which lack proofreading. If we were to copy our large genomes with such error rates this could be catastrophic, but in the context of a virus, if a defective copy is made it is readily replaced.

Viruses, which inhabit their host's cells, reusing the host's own machinery, can also co-opt parts of the host's actual genome into their own. An example is cytomegalovirus (CMV), which infects the majority of the world's population, which has co-opted several immune genes into its own genome and modified them for its own use. Clearly a major driver for such adaptation is to evade the host immune system—viruses in particular use this approach in order to persist long-term within an individual host or a population. The consequence of this is that there has been an extended process of *co-evolution* between hosts and pathogens—the pathogens adapting very quickly, even potentially within days, in a single host in response to an individual's immune response (this is seen in Human Immunodeficiency Virus (HIV), for example).

There is also an important corollary of this in terms of how we understand the immune system—if a pathogen has adapted in order to evade or effectively counter an aspect of the immune response, for example by blocking a chemical signal or an entire cellular pathway, this strongly implicates that particular molecule or pathway in normal strategies of host defence and also defines its limitations. In the same way that hackers can be used by security services to test cyber-defences, studying viruses can teach us a huge amount about the functioning of the normal immune system and how it can be manipulated. Rolf Zinkernagel—whose work with Peter Doherty on how viruses are recognized by lymphocytes led to the Nobel Prize in 1996—describes viruses as 'the best teachers' of immunology (see the Further Reading section at the end of the volume).

Immune systems in different organisms

All organisms have some form of immunity, and the form it takes depends on the environment in which they live and the threats they face. We share many immunologic features with other mammals, which is one reason that the mouse immune system can be used as a reasonable model by immunologists, but sophisticated host defence systems have been in evidence for much longer than this, perhaps around thirty million years.

We might not expect to discover that bacteria—commonly thought of as the invader rather than the host—themselves have an interesting and surprisingly sophisticated form of immunity against infection. Bacteria can suffer invasive threats from specialized viruses, known as *phages*, that are able to hitchhike on the bacterial DNA. Bacteria have learned to defend themselves through the development of a system known as *CRISPR* (clustered, regularly interspaced, short palindromic repeats).

4

This is based on the activity of a family of *Cas* molecules (e.g. Cas9), which can create breaks in, or 'nick', DNA in order to interrupt its sequence and effectively eliminate the gene. These nicking molecules need to be guided in order to do this or they would end up disrupting important host genes. However, they can do so according to a specific set of nucleic acid guides—generated from CRISPR DNA sequences—which target the sites of invasion. This allows the bacteria to police their own DNA sequences effectively and respond to invasive genes.

What makes this system sophisticated is that bacteria will deliberately capture foreign DNA sequences in the CRISPR regions in order to target specific phages and thus they adapt their immune system (see Figure 1). These steps of *recognition* of infection, followed by host modifications leading to a *specific response* and *long-term memory* in the organism are mirrored in the human immune system, although multiple different recognition strategies are used and multiple cells are involved in the response.

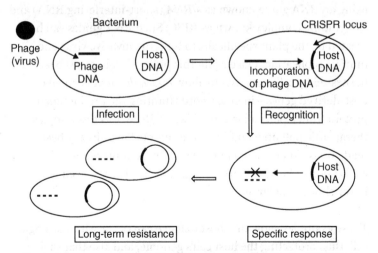

1. **Bacteria can respond specifically to viruses through the CRISPR/ Cas system, which creates a modified copy of the virus sequence (shown as a dotted line) that the cell can use to destroy the invading phage.**

While this sounds interesting enough as a mechanism for bacterial host defence, the system can be harnessed for our own use in molecular biology. By introducing this system into mammalian cells, and directing it using CRISPR guides designed towards genes of interest, we can disrupt or repair genomes very efficiently. The discovery of CRISPR/Cas is only very recent—but it is already having a huge impact in a field known as *genome editing* with enormous scientific and potentially therapeutic potential: we may in time be able to edit human genomes. Interestingly, viruses may have got here first—*mimiviruses*, which are giant viruses with complex genomes, have been found to show signs of a CRISPR-like system to protect themselves against their own viruses (*virophages*).

Plants, too, are susceptible to viruses in the same way that animals and bacteria are and they have their own system of defence. RNA viruses in plants can be degraded by a process known as *RNA interference*. Targeting this process to the invasive RNA rather than the host's own RNA is achieved, like CRISPR/Cas, by using an RNA guide known as *siRNA* (short-interfering RNA) and a degrading complex known as RISC. Such RNA guides can be created by the plant specifically to bind the invasive virus and limit its replication. Once again this piece of biology has been harnessed by cell biologists to allow *knock down* of particular host-derived genes—in other words limiting the production of protein from a particular gene. Like CRISPR/Cas this also has therapeutic potential and various attempts have already been made to use knock down in humans, for example to limit the replication of hepatitis viruses and cancer cells, and even to lower cholesterol levels.

These examples show that host defence can occur within a single cell, thus protecting the host cell's genome, and also that such mechanisms can be of huge significance to human biology, even if they are not part of our own immune system.

Other mechanisms that have a long evolutionary history have been maintained as a critical component of human immunity. For example, *Toll* receptors were originally identified in fruit flies by Nüsslein-Volhard and Wieschaus (*Toll* is German for 'amazing'—apparently this was exclaimed on their discovery). They play an important role in the development of the insect embryo, but later were discovered to also initiate its immune responses against fungi, through the release of anti-microbial proteins and activation of immune cells. Humans possess a similar array of related proteins named '*Toll*-like receptors', which signal and activate immune responses. Although the downstream consequences are more complex in terms of the diversity of cells activated, the initiation process is remarkably similar to that found in the fruit fly (this is discussed further in Chapter 2).

Such pattern recognition and induction of anti-microbial defence is common in many organisms, but the development of immune responses which show classical adaptive features—generation of highly diverse responses which are specific for individual pathogens—does not occur until later in evolution (although CRISPR/Cas may be considered an exception). The first example of an immune system that is most like that seen in a human is the jawless fish (e.g. the lamprey). These animals possess a mechanism for generating pathogen-specific receptors which is parallel to, but distinct from, the one we use as humans (see Chapter 3). Interestingly they also create soluble versions of these receptors which are equivalent to our own antibodies, as well as cell-bound versions, which are more like our own T lymphocytes. From the jawed fish onwards, the evolution of an obvious immune system can be seen.

The human immune system

The immune system is not limited to a single set of specialized cells with discrete functions, but is embedded in every cell in the body.

When considering the human immune system, therefore, it is important not to neglect the role of tissues which immunologists did not generally consider to be 'immunological' (see Figure 2). The skin for example plays a special role in host defence against bacteria and viruses. For viruses, which require a live cell for replication, the presence of a dead cell layer at the skin's outer surface represents a 'wall of death' preventing ready access for many infections. Only some viruses, such as human papilloma viruses, which can cause benign warts as well, leading to the development of cancers such as cervical cancer, are able to infect cells in the skin, but these are at deeper layers. The skin also provides bacterial protection, for example through the secretion of antimicrobial fatty acids. Skin defects are readily accompanied by the development of bacterial infections locally—burns patients in particular are highly susceptible.

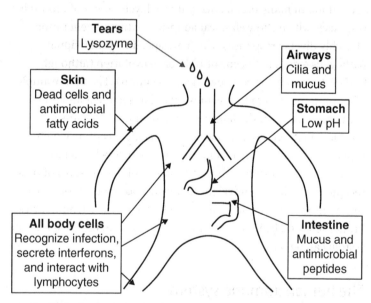

2. **All cells in the body contribute to immunity through their ability to sense infection. Additionally there are discrete structures that form critical barriers at interfaces, with further structures that belong clearly to the immune system itself.**

Nevertheless, despite the host's best efforts to create an unattractive surface environment, what is really achieved at the skin's surface is a relatively peaceful coexistence with multiple micro-organisms. Some of these can cause serious disease at other sites—for example, *Staphylococcus aureus* is a feared invasive bacterium which can create severe tissue damage in many body organs, but it is carried harmlessly by around one in four of us at the entrance to our nostrils. Other Staphyloccal species (e.g. *Staphylococcus epidermidis* or coagulase negative staphylococci) possess a less fearsome armoury of invasive genes, and are major colonizers of the skin in all of us from birth onwards. Even these 'commensals', however, can set up serious infection if the skin's barrier is breached, giving them access to other sites (e.g. the same adherence properties which allow them to colonize the skin can also help them set up long-term infection on plastic artificial joints and heart valves). The eye possesses its own specialized defence system to protect the cornea—tears contain an enzyme called lysozyme (one of the first antimicrobial molecules discovered by Alexander Fleming, who later discovered penicillin). Lysozyme binds to and destroys many bacteria.

The skin represents a huge outer barrier to potential pathogens, but surface immunology also continues within the body's interior. The upper respiratory tract and lungs are major sites of infection and all those reading this book will be familiar with the consequences of rhinovirus infections which cause the common cold. Unlike the skin, where a multi-layered barrier can be developed with clear physical protective qualities, these areas are protected only with a thin *mucous membrane*. In particular, in the lungs, the lining cells (or epithelia) are very thin in order to allow gas exchange. One immune feature of the respiratory tract mediated by physical structures is the so-called ciliary 'escalator', where the epithelial cells possess tiny hair-like structures (cilia) which beat as a group and together lead to the continuous movement of the mucus lining the airways up and out of the lungs. Thus invasive organisms such as bacteria are

9

trapped in the mucus and continuously swept away from sensitive sites into the upper respiratory tract where they are relatively harmless.

The contents of the upper respiratory tract, like the skin, are typically far from sterile. Our throats contain many potentially dangerous bacteria such as the pneumococcus, which is a major cause of pneumonia if allowed to invade lung tissue. The importance of the ciliary escalator is seen in a rare set of diseases (ciliary syndromes) where their function is genetically impaired. Loss of ciliary defence leads to the development of chronic lung disease caused by bacteria (leading to *bronchiectasis*—destruction of lung tissue). Another genetic disease which affects the muco-ciliary escalator is cystic fibrosis (CF). Here there is a defect in the cellular pumps which form mucus, leading to the mucus becoming excessively sticky and thick. As a result, individuals who have the CF genetic defect are prone to recurrent bacterial infections of the lung.

Mucosal defence continues below the diaphragm where, if anything, the stakes are even higher for the host. The gut contains trillions of bacteria—indeed 90 per cent of the cells within the human body are thought to be bacterial. This complex flora or *microbiome* is held at bay by the thin epithelium of the gut, again accompanied by its own mucus layer. These bacteria can cause serious disease if they cross this membrane, as is evident if the bowel is perforated. Limiting the immune response to normal gut contents, while being able to resist invasion by disease-causing micro-organisms, is a delicate balance in the gut, which will be discussed further in Chapter 6. In the upper gut, stomach acid, secreted by specialized cells, serves as an important antimicrobial defence mechanism. Neutralization of this acid makes infection easier for ingested organisms. Other hidden but important immune defence mechanisms are contained within other gut secretions such as, saliva, bile, and a thin layer of mucus in the large bowel.

Beyond these specific structures, all cells possess mechanisms to recognize when they are infected (we will discuss these further in Chapter 2). These mechanisms may trigger the death of that cell, so that an infection cannot spread, as well as secretions giving critical signals to both restrict the growth of viruses and bacteria and to alert and recruit other immune cells. The most important of these are *interferons*, discussed further in Chapter 2.

Specific structures in the immune system

In addition to these basic mechanisms of immunity, the more complex activities of the immune system possess their own structure, although it is diffusely spread (see Figure 3). The critical cells—*white blood cells* or leukocytes—are generated in the bone marrow, along with red blood cells and platelets. The leukocyte subsets are highly diverse, each with their own specialist functions, but they are broadly divided into *myeloid* (which develop in the marrow) and *lymphoid* (which develop in lymphoid structures) leukocytes. The lymphoid structures include the thymus, the lymph nodes, and the spleen. The myeloid cells will be dealt with further in Chapter 2 but, briefly, they exit the marrow fully formed and transit through the body able to respond to infection and tissue damage wherever they find it. In contrast, many lymphoid cells require a period of education, and while they can also effectively survey the whole body, long-term they often find their niche back in specialized tissues.

The thymus lies in the central part of the chest, just behind the sternum and indeed is sometimes removed by surgeons who open the sternum during chest surgery in order to access the tissues behind. It is most prominent in children, consistent with the period of major development of the immune system, but later it becomes quite atrophied, replaced by fat in adulthood and old age. A thymus is required for the development of *T cells*—indeed the name 'T cell' means 'thymus-derived', in contrast to *B cells*, which develop in the Bursa of Fabricius in birds and the bone marrow in

11

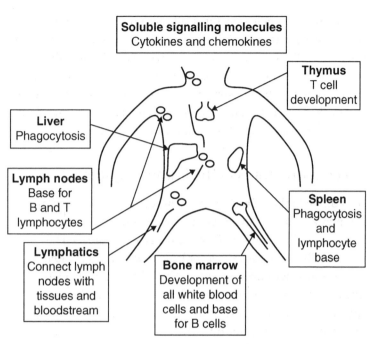

Soluble signalling molecules
Cytokines and chemokines

Thymus
T cell
development

Liver
Phagocytosis

Lymph nodes
Base for
B and T
lymphocytes

Spleen
Phagocytosis
and
lymphocyte
base

Lymphatics
Connect lymph
nodes with
tissues and
bloodstream

Bone marrow
Development of
all white blood
cells and base
for B cells

3. A number of immunological anatomical structures are critical for the development and normal functioning of the immune system.

mammals. The exact educational process within the thymus will be explored further in Chapter 3, but its importance can be gauged by the dramatic impact of failure to generate this organ. The thymus is derived embryologically from the *branchial arches*—evolutionarily ancient, gill-like structures in the neck region which also develop into the inner ear and jaw. In certain congenital defects (e.g. DiGeorge syndrome) these arches do not develop properly, meaning babies are born without a thymus and, therefore, they lack a properly formed T cell compartment, which leaves them with a major susceptibility to infection. Interestingly, this can now be treated by the use of a *thymic transplant* (thymus tissue inserted under the skin), which is able to support T cell development and so reduce the risk of infection.

T cells and B cells may be found in any tissue but their natural first home is in lymphoid tissue. Lymph nodes develop at distinctive sites within the body, for example there are distinct clusters in the neck, armpits, and groin, which can be felt as small, rounded, mobile structures. Lymphocytes are able to access this tissue through specialized venules, using specific cell surface receptors to gain access and in response to chemical 'find-me' cues, released by the node itself. Lymphocytes which have been matured in the bone marrow and thymus but have not yet encountered a specific infection (i.e. *naive* lymphocytes) will typically reside in the lymphatic organs long-term. Similarly, those cells that have responded to an infection and, as a consequence, are forming long-term memory (see Chapter 4), will likewise return there. Across many different animals, including humans, lymph nodes therefore hold a special place in initiating and sustaining immune responses. For example, mice which lack signals to generate lymph nodes (e.g. mice engineered to have a mutation in Lymphotoxin receptor genes) have a severe immune deficiency.

The lymph nodes are supplied by blood as described earlier, but they have another important input—lymph. Lymph is fluid which is derived from the body's tissues generally, carried by thin, narrow, vein-like structures. It can be viewed as a *filtrate* of the plasma in the blood—forced out of the blood vessels by the circulatory system pressure, but containing no red blood cells. Lymph provides an important source of information for the immune system about the status of tissues, carrying cells and proteins to the node for sampling and, if needed, a rapid immune response. The flux of lymph is critical not only for lymph node function but also for normal control of body fluid balance. In situations where the lymphatics are damaged—such as in the disease filariasis, caused by helminth (a worm) infection, or following surgery or radiotherapy for treatment of cancer—chronic accumulation of fluid can occur leading to limb swelling: a condition termed *lymphoedema*.

While the lymph nodes constantly act to survey the lymph and hence the tissues, the spleen offers another important site for lymphocyte development, only its role in surveillance includes the whole bloodstream. The spleen, which lies on the left-hand side of the abdomen, tucked under the ribs, was in the past under-recognized as an immunologic organ. However, it plays a major role in the uptake of bacteria and the clearance of infection. This is very obvious in individuals who lack a spleen—for example, if it needs to be surgically removed following abdominal trauma. Such people are at very great risk of infection by specific bacteria (particularly those possessing a capsule such as the pneumococcus) and require vaccinations as well as, often, preventive antibiotics to minimize the risk of overwhelming infection. This clearance function is not carried out by lymphocytes but rather by specialized myeloid cells (*macrophages*), termed *phagocytes* (i.e. eating cells), that can engulf blood-borne bacteria in the slow flow of the spleen. As a result, in chronic or recurrent infections such as malaria, the spleen can become massively enlarged in size.

The other major site where such phagocyte activity is crucial is the liver. Here specialized macrophages called *Kupffer cells* remove bacteria from the venous blood leaving the gut, thus providing a further protective firewall.

To describe the immune system in terms of these structures alone—important as they are—would, however, miss a crucial point, which is that this system is highly connected and integrated, containing many soluble and therefore invisible components. The primary immune cell types (myeloid and lymphoid compartments) have already been discussed, but they function by communicating using a series of signalling molecules which they can secrete and then sense. Soluble signalling molecules known as *cytokines* provide information about how the immune response cells should react; they are signals to effect growth; and they can act as effector molecules to boost antiviral defence (e.g. interferons, see Chapter 2).

Chemokines are a specialized group of soluble chemicals that aid in the positioning of immune cells, drawing them to lymphoid organs or sites of infection, for example. These small molecules are usually secreted from one cell and form a gradient in the affected tissues to attract the required immune cells. Knowledge of such soluble transmitters of immunologic information are increasingly important as we develop sophisticated methods for blocking them individually in order to modulate the immune system in cases where they are malfunctioning.

One of the best-established aspects of the immune system which has no physical structure at all is the *complement system*, which we will deal with in Chapter 2. This provides a mechanism not only to sense micro-organisms and tissue damage, but also to respond directly, for example by binding to the bacteria and killing them.

Thus the immune system can be considered to be represented by the whole body—each cell in the body has its own internal immune response mechanisms; and there are specialist structures in organs to limit infection. Surveying and integrating these cellular responses, there sits a more specialized or 'professional' team of immune cells with their designated structures for cell education and development, and between the two a series of soluble mediators and mobile cells are in continuous communication.

The immune system has been described as a 'floating brain', and the parallel with the nervous system is apt. Both must respond to diverse internal and external cues, and both must 'learn' in addition to following preset behaviours. The distinction between behaviours which we are born with (i.e. *innate*) and those which we must learn is obvious in the nervous system (e.g. innate: breathing, responding to pain; learned: acquiring language, musical and sports skills). Different components of the brain are responsible for these specialized activities.

This broad split is also very well established in the immune system. There are a set of innate responses which we are born with, and which can respond immediately and effectively to infections generally. This is coupled closely with *adaptive* immunity, which encompasses learned and very specific responses to individual infections. Innate immunity represents the initial immune response and may be sufficient to protect an individual against an immediate threat. The adaptive immune system, being more complex and specific, takes longer to respond to threats the first time, but has a quality—like the brain—of memory, based on specific infections inducing populations of lymphocytes (memory B and T cells). In Chapter 2 we will investigate how the very first responses are triggered and how the immune system possesses senses very similar to those of the brain.

Chapter 2
First responders: the innate immune response

Every immune response has to start somewhere—but how does the system know when to respond? This fundamental question has occupied immunologists for decades, as it is central to understanding both normal responses (e.g. to infections) and abnormal responses (e.g. in auto-immune diseases), as well as in designing vaccines and new therapies for cancer and infectious diseases. In this chapter we will look at how the first triggers are pulled and how important these initial interactions are.

For many years, the central paradigm of the immune system was its ability to distinguish self from non-self. In other words, the presence of self led to no response, whereas the presence of something different—a transplanted organ, for example—would trigger a response. The focus was on how the immune system recognizes *antigens*—specific structures derived from biologic molecules such as proteins. Over the last twenty-five years, however, our knowledge has developed, as it has become evident that it is not just the antigen itself, but the context in which it is presented, that is important. One theory proposed by Polly Matzinger in the 1990s was that of *danger*. If a new antigen is encountered in the presence of additional signals indicating it as being dangerous, then a functional immune response is induced.

The big breakthrough in this area came with the discovery of how such a danger could be sensed; the idea of the immune system being very sensitive to *pathogen-associated molecular patterns* (PAMPs) having already been proposed by Charles (Charlie) Janeway some years previously. These PAMPs are predictable features common to micro-organisms but distinct from their hosts. The breakthrough came with the discovery of multiple families of such receptors that have evolved to 'sense' pathogens, fully confirming Janeway's theory. Finely tuned recognition of such PAMPs kick-starts a host's defence against the specific pathogens, driving much of what happens later in the immune response.

This process has been found to be even more extensive, to include the idea of *damage-associated molecular patterns* or DAMPs. These are signals that are present in damaged but not healthy tissue—for example, with cell contents being released into the surrounding area upon cell injury. The related nature of the sensing of PAMPs and DAMPs explains why similar patterns of immune response can be seen in the cases of tissue damage as well as in infection.

Sensing danger

The ability to sense PAMPs is not present in all cells. Even within the specialized cells of the innate immune system, some subsets possess a more effective armoury than others in this regard. These cells include an important set derived from the myeloid compartment (see Figure 4). The *monocytes* are an abundant subset of cells which circulate in the blood and are able to migrate into tissues, where they convert into macrophages—the phagocytic cells we already encountered in the spleen. Monocytes also convert into a set of cells known as *dendritic* cells, which were for a long time ignored but have since been found to hold a central position in the immune system. Dendritic cells possess, as can be seen in Figure 4, a wavy and involuted surface (they were previously

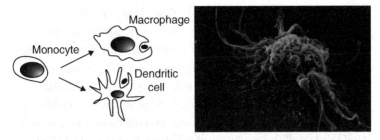

4. Macrophages and dendritic cells, which belong to the myeloid lineage, are phagocytic cells, derived from monocytes, which circulate in the blood. The electron micrograph shows a dendritic cell.

known as *veiled cells*) and an array of PAMP sensors situated so they can recognize particular molecules that they encounter or take up. These cells are thus able to sense danger using multiple sensors, and once sensed, effectively coordinate an immune response from that point on.

Bacteria possess an array of common PAMPs which can be sensed by host cells. One especially potent example is a molecule known as LPS (lipopolysaccharide) which is part of the outer membrane of many bacterial species, particularly so-called *Gram negative* bacteria. (Hans Christian Gram published stains of these bacteria over a century ago for bacterial classification and they are still routinely used.) LPS is sensed, even at extremely low concentrations, by the immune system through a Toll-like receptor (TLR; in this case TLR4). Activation of TLR4 is an effective danger signal which activates the dendritic cell to secrete cytokines; recruits further immune cells; and initiates a set of widespread responses. If these prove effective in controlling the infection then the LPS disappears and the system returns quickly to normal. In situations where bacteria are very widespread, such as in sepsis due to *Meningococcus*, then responses to LPS can over-activate the immune system with deleterious consequences.

LPS is not the only microbial product the body can sense. Indeed, TLR4 itself is also able to recognize a lipid generated by malarial parasites. Other parts of bacterial cell walls can be sensed by further Toll-like receptors (e.g. TLR2 is important in the sensing of *Mycobacterium tuberculosis* (Mtb), the agent causing tuberculosis (TB)). These receptors lie at the cell surface, where they can survey the extracellular environment. Other similar receptors lie within the cell, assessing engulfed or intracellular PAMPs (that is, PAMPs derived from organisms infecting the cell itself). Intracellular receptors of a distinct type such as *NOD2* (nucleotide-binding oligomerization domain-containing protein 2) can recognize specific components of Gram-positive bacteria. NOD2 is of some interest because the gene encoding this protein is polymorphic—that is, it varies between individuals (this is explored in more detail in Chapter 5). Some variants of the gene are linked with protection against *Mycobacterium leprae*, the bacterium which causes leprosy. Variations in NOD2 are also strongly associated with the development of inflammatory bowel disease, potentially through modifying how bacteria in the gut are handled. It is thought that where there is redundancy or backup in the system, the large team of sensors is able to cope against different threats (NOD2 itself may be able to sense viruses, for example)—but that individual receptors can still play a dominant role in protection against infection and the development of disease.

Viruses, which hijack cellular machinery to replicate within cells they have infected, also generate unique danger signals. When RNA viruses, like influenza, replicate, they generate double-stranded RNA—a form of RNA that does not exist in healthy host cells. Consequently, a number of alarm systems develop in the host to recognize these double-stranded RNA (e.g. one using the protein RIG-I; see Figure 2) and again, like those for the recognition of LPS, they are remarkably sensitive. This sensitivity is important as viruses generally replicate very fast, making fast reaction times crucial in mounting a response before the host is overwhelmed. However, some viruses, such as the Hepatitis C Virus (HCV), have evolved mechanisms to disrupt this signalling in order to gain the advantage. RNA derived from HCV can be sensed in an infected liver cell through RIG-I, but HCV then produces a molecule which specifically interrupts the signalling, thus preventing the initiation of an effective antiviral response.

Dangerous DNA can also be sensed. Whereas, in human DNA, certain types of sequences are chemically modified via a process known as *methylation*, in bacteria these same types of sequences are not and so they can be recognized by the Toll-like receptor TLR9, which initiates an immune response. Similarly, whereas mammalian DNA is contained within the nucleus, viral DNA is present outside the nucleus and so can be detected by a recently discovered pathway that includes the use of two critical molecules, CGAS and STING. The sensor CGAS normally exists as a series of isolated molecules in the cell, which are inactive on their own. However, if foreign DNA is present, this binds them together, creating a multi-unit enzyme which produces a small molecule called cyclic GMP. This then transmits a signal to STING, which in turn leads to the generation of interferons by the cell (see Figure 2).

These are several examples of danger-sensing mechanisms that function as alarm bells in the immune system. Overall they are described as innate mechanisms, being an inherently active part of a healthy organism and not requiring prior exposure to the pathogens concerned in order to be able to respond when needed (see Figure 5).

Responding to danger

The immune system having been alerted, it is important that rapid action is taken to limit the spread of the pathogen. A number of responses can be initiated immediately and these also form a critical part of innate immunity. Overall this group of responses contributes to what has long been recognized as *inflammation*, the local accumulation of activated cells in tissues responding to tissue injury.

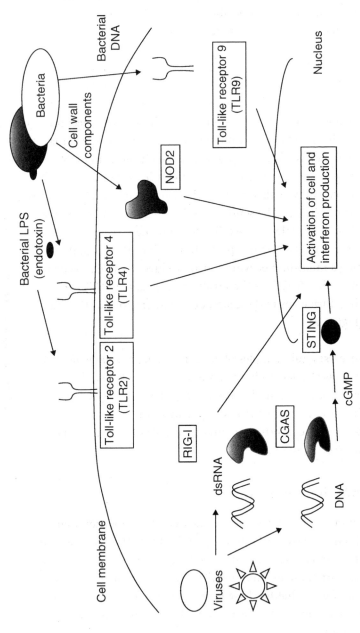

5. Mechanisms for sensing danger include recognition of double-stranded RNA within a cell, sensed by RIG-1, DNA within the cell cytoplasm, sensed by CGAS, and other viral and bacterial ligands, sensed by Toll-like receptors.

An important set of early responses are mediated by the interferon system. Interferons were discovered half a century ago as elements that limited virus replication, and over time their central role in host defence has been firmly cemented. Animals with mutations limiting interferon signalling are highly susceptible to virus infections. So-called Type I interferons (alpha and beta) can be generated by most cells, and most cells also possess receptors for these molecules. A signal from interferon alpha induces an astonishing array of responses within a cell, with many hundreds of genes being upregulated. This includes genes which can shut down virus replication, for example by degrading RNA within the cell and limiting protein production. They also play an important role in instructing the adaptive immune response and generating effective immunity over time.

Interferons can also be used therapeutically, for example in the treatment of chronic Hepatitis B Virus (HBV) and HCV, although they are only partially effective—because the viruses have already adapted to deal with the natural interferon responses induced within the host. For HCV a different interferon system—interferon lambda—appears to be important. Individuals with specific versions of the interferon lambda 3 gene are up to five times more likely to clear this virus after exposure, and thus avoid chronic infection and liver disease.

Viruses are intracellular parasites and thus mechanisms to control them are focused on the infected cells. In contrast, bacteria more typically replicate outside cells and require different immune responses. One of these is to bring in a major subset of innate immune cells known as *neutrophils*. Neutrophils are myeloid cells with a multi-lobed nucleus and a very granular cytoplasm. These, together with related cells called *eosinophils* and *basophils* are collectively known as *granulocytes* and polymorphonuclear cells or *polymorphs*. Neutrophils are important in bacterial and also fungal defence—loss of neutrophils, for example through suppression of their development in bone marrow by drugs used to treat cancers, puts individuals at high risk of severe bacterial infections. They mediate their effects through engulfing micro-organisms (a process known as *phagocytosis*), followed by the generation of toxic mediators derived from hydrogen peroxide (effectively, a form of biological bleach), and through release of their granules, which contain antibacterial molecules. Phagocytosis is a critical step in host defence and once micro-organisms are taken into the neutrophil, they are subsequently destroyed by digestion in specialized compartments within these cells that contain highly active enzymes (*lysosomes*).

Neutrophils do not live for long in normal circumstances, just a few days, and in the context of an acute response to infection, they die 'on the battlefield'. But before they do so there is one final act—extrusion of their nuclei. This forms a *NET* (neutrophil extracellular trap) from the long strands of DNA in the nucleus, rather like a spider's web that can capture bacteria and enhance their clearance. Related granulocytes—*eosinophils* and *basophils*—are involved in a distinct type of immune response, particularly that triggered by worm infections. These cells, together with their companion T cells and tissue-resident *mast cells* involved in such responses, are discussed further in Chapter 6.

Neutrophil activity can be damaging to the host and thus needs some direction in order to attract the immune response to the area of infection and to organize its function. One important orchestrator of this is the *complement system*. Complement is an essential component of the immune system that is made in the liver and then circulates in the bloodstream. Here it functions as a complex team of proteins, a so-called *cascade*, whereby a small signal can become massively amplified locally as it progresses by activating other members of the family sequentially. The complement cascade can be activated initially by different means, including the binding of antibodies. However, it can also be activated through direct encounter with a microbe or with innate danger signals such as those from tissue damage to immediately liberate active components which bind to the bacteria and attract neutrophils. Bacteria which have been decorated with complement components, or *opsonized*, are easier for phagocytes to take up and destroy. Other complement components can bind to bacteria to create pores in their membrane and thereby destroy them. Their particular importance as antibacterial molecules is evident in families with defects in these 'terminal' complement proteins—these are at increased risk of infections with invasive bacteria such as *Meningococcus*.

The complement system in humans is highly evolved and complex, with around thirty proteins linking innate and adaptive immunity in a tightly regulated fashion (see Figure 6)—and the complement system itself is evolutionarily very ancient, probably over 500 million years old. Complement components are found in cnidarians—jellyfish and sea anemones—where the system plays a role in host defence as well as the inflammatory response.

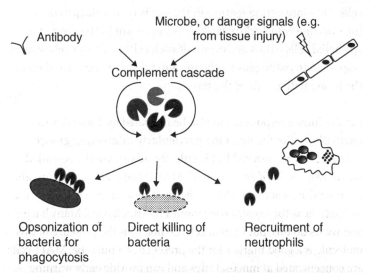

Antibody

Microbe, or danger signals (e.g. from tissue injury)

Complement cascade

Opsonization of bacteria for phagocytosis

Direct killing of bacteria

Recruitment of neutrophils

6. **Complement proteins can be activated by antibodies, microbes, or innate danger signals (e.g. from tissue injury). Once activated, a 'cascade' occurs which leads to activation of more complement components and massive amplification of the signal.**

The innate response is not only the preserve of the phagocytes. Lymphocytes can also play a role as exemplified by the activity of *natural killer* (NK) cells. NK cells are derived from bone marrow but do not require maturation in the thymus; they feature a set of receptors which respond to stress signals and virus infection. NK cells can either kill the cell, by releasing a set of toxic granules; or they can release interferons, which suppress viral replication. NK cells can also sense danger—they possess receptors which can be triggered by the expression of specific stress signals on a cell's surface and also recognize 'missing self', which is the removal of cell surface proteins by viruses in an attempt to hide.

A further group of lymphoid cells which are related to NK cells and have only recently been uncovered are the *innate lymphoid cells* (ILCs), which are a rare but potent subset of immune cells. Found in tissues, they appear to play an important role in initiating and controlling inflammation. They are potent secretors of cytokines and thus can direct the effector functions of many other cells. One interesting feature in the gut is their ability to make the cytokine Interleukin 22. This is important in the growth of epithelial cells—thus activation of such cells not only orchestrates responses to pathogens by the immune response but also directs the immediate repair of the tissue.

Finally, innate responses can also be mediated by T and B cells, particularly the former. One particularly interesting group, only recently discovered but highly abundant, are the so-called *mucosal-associated invariant T* (MAIT) cells. These cells are able to recognize a bacterial PAMP—in this case a small molecule made by bacteria as they synthesize vitamin B2 (riboflavin). Many bacteria and yeasts do this, but human cells do not, thus the presence of this molecule is a good marker for the presence of a microbe. MAIT cells are concentrated at mucosal sites and can provide early warning and immediate effector functions in host defence. They are just one example of what may be called a *bridging* population—a set of cells which possess both innate and adaptive characteristics.

The acute phase response

So far we have considered the molecules and cells involved in the first responses to infection. In thinking about the whole organism these responses are integrated and produce not only local effects (inflammation) but also major changes in physiology (see Figure 7). The secretion of soluble mediators like cytokines and interferons means the activity can be spread throughout the body, as these signalling molecules can act at a distance. For example, the liver will, in response to the cytokines induced by bacterial infection, secrete several proteins which aid the host immune response. It will signal to shut down iron stores and limit access to iron for bacteria—which require this for replication. It also secretes a

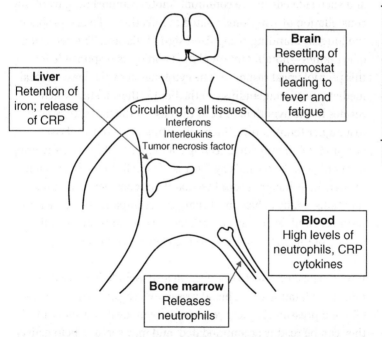

Liver
Retention of iron; release of CRP

Circulating to all tissues
Interferons
Interleukins
Tumor necrosis factor

Brain
Resetting of thermostat leading to fever and fatigue

Blood
High levels of neutrophils, CRP cytokines

Bone marrow
Releases neutrophils

7. **The acute phase response to infection results from the sensing of danger and leads to multiple effects throughout the body, mostly mediated by circulating soluble mediators such as interferons and other cytokines.**

molecule called *C reactive protein* (CRP), which like complement can opsonize bacteria for phagocytosis. Measurement of CRP in the bloodstream is an indicator of bacterial infection and is widely used in clinical medicine. A similar robust response which is clinically used is measurement of the neutrophil count in blood (released from the bone marrow), which goes up markedly in the acute phase response—typically in bacterial rather than viral infections.

Interferons have many effects on the body, including changes in appetite and induction of fatigue (so-called 'sickness behaviour'). Many of the symptoms we regard as flu-like are in fact mediated by the interferon response—this is particularly evident when interferons are used therapeutically (e.g. to treat viral hepatitis), and such side effects are common. Another important part of this constellation of symptoms related to infection is fever—probably the longest-standing recognized sign of disease. The secretion of cytokines—notably Interleukins 1 and 6—is responsible for this physiological response. The cytokines act via release of local mediators (prostaglandins) on the body's 'thermostat' which resides in the hypothalamus, at the base of the brain, to reset it to a higher temperature. Such a resetting leads to the classic symptom of an individual feeling cold and possibly even shivering but being hot to touch. Why fever is of benefit to the host is not fully clear, although it could be that it enhances some immune functions. Many behavioural changes accompany the acute phase response, and fever may potentially serve to limit the overall impact of infection, or even its spread between hosts.

Physiological responses to infection also include increased heart rate and dilatation of the blood vessels, which can lead to lowering of blood pressure. If these responses are modest and short-lived they can be readily accommodated, and may serve to help deliver oxygen to tissues. However, more severe infections can lead to quite exaggerated responses and reduced blood pressure can be life-threatening, inducing a state known as *septic shock*. Even once the infection has been treated with antibiotics, the cascade of cytokines can continue to sustain this abnormal physiological state, which may require a person to require additional support in an intensive care unit to monitor and moderate blood pressure levels and the function of organs such as the lungs and kidneys.

Innate responses are tuned to sense very small local signals, and thus recognize danger early. However, their effects may be systemic, also acting on the bone marrow to release more neutrophils (so-called *emergency granulopoesis*); on the brain to change behaviour and reset temperature; and on blood vessels to change blood delivery. The responses therefore include concurrently some of the most subtle and some of the most dramatic features of the immune system. Perhaps because of these rather pronounced and well-recognized changes, the innate response used to be regarded as relatively unsophisticated and stereotypical, but as more is learned about it, its complexity becomes increasingly evident.

These immune responses are highly evolved in sensing pathogens, and so, of course, pathogens have in turn evolved to evade them. Harnessing the body's innate response is the focus of vaccine development and immunotherapy—one effective treatment for warts (human papillomavirus) is a TLR7 agonist cream and soluble TLR agonists are on trial for the treatment of viral hepatitis. One final development in our knowledge is that rather than simply finding that innate responses only act early and adaptive immune responses later, very often the two processes have been found to be acting in concert. Innate mechanisms are enhanced by adaptive responses (antibodies activate complement and opsonize bacteria for phagocytosis), while adaptive responses harness innate effectors (e.g. T cells recruiting neutrophils and eosinophils). This continued activity means that blocking the innate response can also be of enormous value in chronic inflammatory diseases—where such pathways are aberrantly and persistently activated. We will revisit this idea in Chapter 7.

Chapter 3
Adaptive immunity: a voyage of (non-)self-discovery

A key question addressed in this chapter is how the immune system can respond to so many diverse threats—including viruses (e.g. the severe respiratory infections SARS and MERS Co-V) that we have never encountered previously as a species. This inherent diversity in the immune system can be explained by analysis of how the adaptive immune system is put together—in particular the receptors on B and T lymphocytes.

B cells and antibodies

B cells are lymphocytes that develop in the bone marrow and are able to secrete antibodies for immunologic protection. Antibodies are highly specialized proteins that are able to bind to a particular target (e.g. the outer coat of a bacterium or virus), known as an *antigen* or *epitope*. Following binding this can lead to blocking of infection (*neutralization*), activation of the complement system, and uptake by phagocytes. If the antigen is on the surface of a cell (say, an infected cell or a cancer cell), it can lead to the killing of that cell. A vast range of antibodies can be produced and this ability to create a broad repertoire is essential—defects in antibody development leave individuals at risk of infection from viruses and bacteria, and indeed from cancer as well. The huge breadth of the antibody repertoire stems from the mechanisms used to make antibodies, which, although encoded in the genome like all other genes, undergo some particular tricks to create diversity.

Antibody (or immunoglobulin) genes are not created as a single unit—if this were the case we would have to inherit a huge number of closely related genes, and even this would carry the risk that it would not cover an individual threat. What is done instead is to stitch genes together from smaller parts, each of which is itself diverse, but which create many more possibilities through various combinations (see Figure 8). Each antibody is made up of two chains, a heavy and a light chain, and it is typically the combination of these chains which provide the specificity—in other words, the particular capacity to bind one individual target, for example this year's influenza strain but not last year's. The most specific piece of the immunoglobulin heavy chain gene is stitched together (or *recombined*) within the genome of a given B cell, from three types

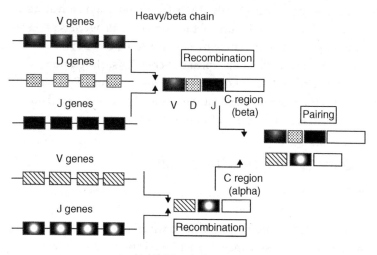

8. The DNA for an antigen receptor or antibody is made up of separate segments which are recombined. These are expressed as *heavy* and *light* chains, which pair together. The process of building a T cell receptor is analogous, except that *alpha* and *beta* chains are used.

of subunit—V, D, and J. Each of these is represented in the genome, side by side, multiple times (44 V, 27 D, and 6 J). Such segments can be combined more or less randomly to provide thousands of possible templates for antibody production. In fact, there is an additional level of diversity introduced as the joining process may introduce additional nucleotides (so-called *junctional diversification*), which can further modify the structure of the antibody at critical sites. A similar process, differing only in the lack of a D segment, occurs on the light chain. In humans, there are actually two different light chain genes, located in two different places in the genome.

Each B cell performs this recombining process independently, and thus as millions of B cells are made, they are able to explore fully the possibilities of combining heavy and light chains to create a very wide set of antibodies for host defence. The process of somatic recombination in B cells is regulated tightly by a number of genes—most importantly RAGs (recombination activating genes), which carefully control this somewhat dangerous process of manipulating and repairing host DNA. Loss of RAGs leaves the host without any means of creating such receptor diversity and thus with no adaptive immune system. Further modifications can be made later to antibodies to improve their effectiveness and 'bolt on' additional functions (see Chapter 4).

T cells: turning cells inside out

B cells create antibodies which can survey the extracellular environment—thus capturing viruses as they infect or spread between cells, or binding to bacteria which live outside of cells. B cells also possess a specific surface receptor, which is a membrane-bound version of the antibody it makes. By binding a soluble (i.e. free-floating) antigen, or a particle such as a virus, this receptor allows the B cell to receive signals about the presence of a target for its receptor. But viruses and other pathogens, including some parasites (e.g. the parasites that cause malaria) and bacteria (e.g. the TB-causing bacterium Mtb mentioned in Chapter 2), live within cells—so how can this internal environment be surveyed? This is the domain of the T cell and its specific sensor, the T cell receptor or TCR. T cells use a similar principle to B cells to create a receptor on their cell surface to interrogate the internal environment of cells.

The basic make-up of a standard-model T cell receptor is very similar to that of a B cell receptor (see Figure 8). The receptor is made of an alpha and beta chain, with similar genes making these up as are found in immunoglobulin heavy and light chains—that is, a palette of V, D, and J regions.

T cells need to sense the internal proteins of a cell—for example, a virus replicating within a target cell. To do this, the immune system has developed a pathway for revealing the protein contents of a cell on the cell surface (see Figure 9). All cells have a mechanism for degrading proteins via the *proteasome*, a complex of protein-cleaving enzymes which form a barrel-shaped organelle. Proteins targeted for degradation are decorated with a small molecule called *ubiquitin*, by a series of enzymes in a tightly regulated process. This includes any proteins made by an invading virus. The ubiquitin-labelled proteins are shuttled to the proteasome where they are cleaved into a variety of lengths of short amino acid sequences—*peptides* or *epitopes*—in the region of ten amino acids long. Such peptides are generated more or less randomly. Some of these peptides are actively pumped into the cell's export compartment, the endoplasmic reticulum, where they encounter the protein used to export them to the cell surface.

The protein used for export is highly evolved for this purpose and is encoded in a critical genetic area for the immune system known as the *Major Histocompatibility Complex* (MHC)—in humans also known as the *Human Leukocyte Antigen* (HLA) complex, or more commonly as the *tissue type*. HLA genes fall into two major classes, Class I and Class II, and in humans there are three major types

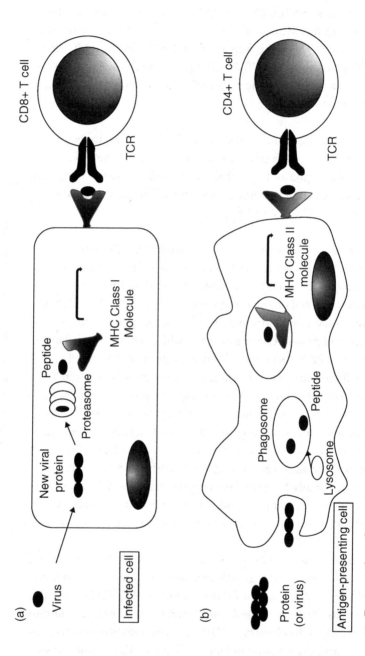

9. Presentation of an antigen (e.g. from a virus) (a) via the MHC Class I pathway to CD8+ T cells; (b) via the MHC Class II pathway, which is a feature of specialized antigen-presenting cells.

34

of Class I proteins: HLA-A, -B, and -C. Each of these molecules is highly adapted for carrying and presenting peptides—they possess a stalk for binding into the cell membrane and then a presenting platform in which there is a groove. Peptides are able to bind tightly into this groove. Thus a fully loaded HLA molecule will possess in its groove a single peptide, bound down tightly and 'visible' to the T cell. It is these peptides which are carefully sensed by the T cells through their receptors.

There is a vast array of possible viruses—and therefore peptides—thus the system of presentation through MHC has to be very flexible. Evolution has solved this problem through the creation of a huge array of different types (*alleles*) of HLA molecules. Across the globe there are more than 3,000 different types of HLA-A molecules and more than 4,000 HLA-B molecules found in humans, making it the most diverse region of the entire human genome. Unlike the B cell and T cell receptors, these do not recombine, and each individual only inherits six such Class I alleles (one set of HLA-A, -B, and -C from each parent). However, so diverse are these, and so many combinations exist, that very few of us have identically matching HLA molecules.

It is this huge diversity within HLA genes that creates a major issue for matching in the setting of organ or bone marrow transplantation, as in this setting, different HLA molecules coming in from the donor can be recognized as foreign, just like a virus, and induce a brisk immune response (see Chapter 6). Indeed, it was this property of providing a barrier to transplantation that first drew immunologists such as Peter Medawar to the MHC as a 'transplantation antigen' before its role in host defence was elucidated by Rolf Zinkernagel and Peter Doherty in the 1970s. The HLA region is the part of the human genome where the effect of evolution is most obvious—it is the most diverse. In other words, developing a wide range of HLAs has been essential for our survival as a species. The likely explanation for this is that it minimizes the chance of a microbe evading T cell responses and sweeping through an entire population. The problems faced by those looking to find matched donors for transplants are therefore a result of a successful evolutionary strategy for defence against severe infection.

Helpers and killers

T cells which are able to respond to peptides bound in the groove of an MHC Class I molecule are described as Class I restricted. They are also characterized by expression of the secondary receptor CD8. CD8 is not only a useful marker for these cells but actually adds to the specificity by also binding very weakly to the MHC molecule and stabilizing the interaction. Once a CD8+ T cell has recognized an infected cell, it is activated to proliferate (thus making more copies of itself and amplifying the response) but also to immediately respond to the threat by killing the target and releasing many signalling molecules—hence they are called *killer* or *cytotoxic* T cells.

There is another major type of T cell response which is involved in coordinating the immune response—the so-called T helper cells. These T cells are characterized by expression of the molecule CD4 on their cell surface and instead of sensing molecules presented by MHC Class I, they use a related system called MHC Class II, which is normally the preserve of a subset of immune cells called 'professional' antigen-presenting cells. The most effective of these cells is the dendritic cell, which has an unrivalled capacity to take up antigens derived from pathogens and present these to the immune system. Dendritic and related cells, such as macrophages, are able to take up, for example, a virus or bacteria, or a part of such a pathogen, into a specialized compartment known as a phagosome. The phagosome then fuses with an organelle called the lysosome. Lysosomal contents are highly acidic and so the pathogen is destroyed and broken down into peptides. These peptides are then immediately loaded onto a Class II molecule, which is then exported to the cell surface (see Figure 9).

Thus while B cells are able to sense and respond to the circulating threats (whole viruses for example), and CD8+ T cells to intracellular threats (viruses in a cell in a tissue), the CD4+ T helper cells sense what is provided for them by the professional antigen-presenting cells such as the dendritic cells. However, although this might appear somewhat limited, the role of CD4+ T cells is absolutely central to the functioning of the immune system, as is evident in the development of AIDS, where CD4+ T cells are lost as they are specifically targeted by HIV. The reason CD4+ T cells are so important is because they can provide help to both CD8+ T cells and B cells, and thus direct their activity. Since they receive their instructions from a highly specialized dendritic cell, they receive not only information about the antigens which are present, but also the context. As already discussed, dendritic cells will also sense the PAMPs associated with a particular infection and provide essential signals to the CD4+ T cell to direct its subsequent response. Since these instructions are given at the earliest stage of an immune response and the CD4+ T cells subsequently conduct the rest of the immunological orchestra as a result, this interaction, and the Class II molecules which direct it, have a major impact on host immunity and its regulation. There are number of different styles of helper T cell, distinguished by the different cytokines they make (e.g. Types 1, 2, and 17), which will be introduced in subsequent chapters as they have important roles in host defence, auto-immunity, and allergy.

Unconventional T cells

There are other T cells with different purposes that fill specific niches. These unconventional T cells differ not only in how they see antigens but also in their role in the immune response, since typically they are infrequently found in the blood but are very much present in the tissues. Here they also partly play the role of first responder seen in Chapter 2. The first such unconventional T cells identified were a T cell subset that, rather than using alpha and beta TCR chains, use a parallel set of receptor chains named gamma and delta, whose target is not the MHC. A series of molecules has been identified which can trigger gamma delta T cells—this includes a bacterial product HMBPP (4-Hydroxy-3-methyl-but-2-enyl pyrophosphate) which appears to function as a very potent ligand. It has been reported that a cell surface molecule, Butyrophilin 3A1, acts as a *presenting molecule* for gamma delta cells. Gamma delta cells are relatively uncommon in human blood but enriched at mucosal sites such as the gut and expand in response to bacterial infections. They are much more common in some other mammals such as sheep, where they may be the dominant type of T cell.

In addition to gamma delta T cells, there are alpha beta T cells with non-MHC specificities. Invariant NK T cells have, as the name suggests, some features of NK cells, but possess a TCR, although they emerge from the thymus with a uniform, distinctive alpha and beta chain. This receptor is able to bind a molecule that is MHC-like, named CD1d, which carries a glycolipid molecule

	Recognizes	Presenting molecule	T cell
	Peptide	MHC	Conventional T cell
	Bacterial metabolite (vitamin)	MR1 (MHC-like)	MAIT cell
	Bacterial metabolite	Butyrophilin	Gamma delta T cell
	Bacterial lipid	CD1d (MHC-like)	Natural killer T (NKT) cell
	Self-lipid in skin	CD1a (MHC-like)	Innate T cell

10. **An increasing number of unconventional T cell subsets have been found which recognize different types of molecules, some of which are similar to MHC molecules but usually not polymorphic (i.e. different between people).**

(i.e. fat- rather than protein-based recognition). One important molecule recognized by these cells is alpha galactosyl-ceramide, which has a combination of a sugar and a lipid molecule derived from bacteria. MAIT cells, mentioned in Chapter 2, are another example—these cells recognize the MHC-related molecule MR1, rather than MHC, presenting a vitamin B2 precursor made by bacteria (but not by humans). These and other unconventional or non-classical T cells are enriched in the liver and the epithelium of the gut in humans. There are likely many other T cell types with alternative recognition strategies to be discovered, probably providing host defence particularly at barrier sites (see Figure 10).

Distribution and recirculation

The lymphocyte subsets created through this process are not distributed randomly through the body but instead are carefully organized anatomically. Such organization is essential for mounting a rapid immune response, as we will discuss in Chapter 4. The CD4+ and CD8+ T cells which leave the thymus have a set of receptors on their surface which gives them specialized access to the lymphoid organs. This occurs through interaction with the blood vessel lining in these tissues organized into so-called high endothelial venules. In contrast they do not have access to normal tissues, even if they are inflamed or infected. The only exception to this rule is the liver, where the endothelium has gaps (*fenestrae* or windows) allowing direct contact between *naive* cells (i.e. cells that have not yet encountered a pathogen) and liver cell populations—a feature which may be relevant to the unique immunology of this organ (see Chapter 5).

Naive T cells can be found in the blood, recirculating between lymph nodes, and are highly concentrated in lymph nodes and the spleen. Naive B cells likewise are concentrated in these regions, which is critical for their biology as they require close interaction with T cells in order to develop into antibody-producing cells. T cells which have been activated are able to leave the lymph nodes, circulate through the blood, and relocate or *home* to tissues throughout the body, providing local defence. They do this by changing the receptors on their cell surface so they no longer bind to the high endothelial venule and instead are attracted to the inflamed endothelium. The unconventional T cells described earlier develop with this tissue-homing programme already in place so they are distributed to tissues directly. This makes sense, as their role is to provide immediate protection and they do not require further education and amplification in the lymph node.

Lymphatics are an important route for travel for lymphocytes as well as other immune cells. Lymphocytes leaving the lymph node do so via small lymphatics, which ultimately drain back into the blood system through the thoracic duct. Once in the blood the naive cells can then recirculate back to the lymph nodes, ensuring the whole range of B and T cell receptors, so carefully created, is well-distributed anatomically to counter diverse incoming threats.

In this chapter, we have seen how an immune system can be constructed to achieve a huge level of diversity from simple building blocks. The drive to do this is enormous—the MHC is the most highly diversified part of the human genome and has been under very strong selection pressure throughout human development. By maintaining a broad array of MHCs in a group, there is less chance of a pathogen overcoming the defences of an individual's or an entire population's immune system—the pathogen must tackle each person afresh. A failure to create MHC diversity would be catastrophic and could lead to an entire population being susceptible to infection.

The theme of diversity is continued and is even more obvious in the antigen receptors on B and T cells. Here the problem has been solved by evolution in a different way, using unique methods of recombination to effectively create millions of extra possible genes for this purpose. In the case of B cells, these genes, and the antibodies that are created from the genetic template, are further honed so they can become highly specific to their target. Effectively the genome of the B cell can be 'trained' to make the best immune response. Thus, while sensitivity and speed are the features of innate immunity discussed in the Chapter 2, diversification and specificity are the parallel features of the adaptive immune response discussed in this chapter. In Chapter 4, we will see how the immune response to such attack is coordinated, and how the potential diversity in attack is put to good use.

Chapter 4
Making memories

So far we have seen how the immune system can sense pathogens generally (e.g. via PAMPs and complement) and how it can target them specifically (e.g. via antibodies secreted from B cells and TCRs on T cells). Clearly all this needs to be tightly coordinated in space—to get the right cells in the right place—but crucially also over time. Let us consider how the response develops following exposure to a virus—following the dictum of Rolf Zinkernagel that viruses are the best teachers of immunology.

Priming the immune response

To make effective *memory*, the immune response needs to be induced correctly, or *primed*, during the initial stages of an infection. The first steps that must be taken by the immune system to develop a response relate to activation of the innate immune system. Without this, as has been established using genetically deficient mice, the adaptive response is subsequently overwhelmed in many cases. Indeed, HCV, which is able to establish chronic infection in most of those infected, is able to suppress and evade the innate immune response for many weeks in order to establish itself. Viruses which invade tissue locally are soon captured by myeloid cells such as macrophages and dendritic cells in order to initiate the innate response. Typically, a virus will present multiple PAMPs, leading to activation of these cells and kick-starting the process of antigen presentation.

Initiating this process in a tissue is of limited value if the aim is to allow presentation to a wide array of naive T cells in the hope of matchmaking the pathogen and its abundant peptide cargo with the appropriate TCR. The dendritic cell needs to relocate to the local lymph node, focusing on the areas where the T cells are concentrated. Here there is a very rapid series of interactions with putative responding T cells in an effort to find a match—in other words, a T cell that can recognize its cargo of MHC-bound peptides. As discussed in Chapter 3, a TCR likely exists for each possible peptide presented on an MHC molecule, although they may only represent one in a million of the normal pool of T cells, so this process must be very efficient, especially because at this point the race is on to develop an immune response as the virus is already replicating rapidly. This phase of the immune response is known as priming.

Once a T cell with the appropriate TCR is identified, the signals to that T cell are very potent and the changes within that cell are profound. One thing that must remain the same is the TCR itself, otherwise the specificity of the response will be lost. Therefore, with the aim of amplifying the response based on this recognition, the first response once such a signal is received is for the cell to proliferate, undergoing a process of cell division to create daughter cells. This proliferative response is enormous—within a few days the T cells responding to a single viral peptide may expand to represent one in ten of the CD8+ T cells in the body. It is also necessary—the T cells need to survey every tissue in the body to seek out and destroy virus-infected cells. The transformation in the T cell is very dramatic and in addition to proliferating, it rapidly acquires characteristics such as the ability to destroy the antigen; to make soluble molecules such as interferon gamma (which shares many antiviral characteristics with interferon alpha), tumor necrosis factor, and chemokines; and to attract other cells. Such cells are known as *effector T cells*, as opposed to the naive cells found pre-infection. CD4+ T cells are also activated and the populations of antiviral CD4+ T cells expand at this time.

Meanwhile a B cell response is also induced—again based in a lymph node. The organization of this B cell response is anatomically discrete—B cells secrete antibodies which can have an effect around the body even though the producing cells may be tightly localized. B cells require help from CD4+ T cells in order to produce fully optimized antibody responses. This activity is concentrated in specialized areas of the lymphoid tissue called *germinal centres* (see Figure 11). Within the sites where the antigen is concentrated B cells compete with each other for signals and space. This is a very effective way of ensuring that—from all the antibodies available—the most effective are amplified rapidly. Within the

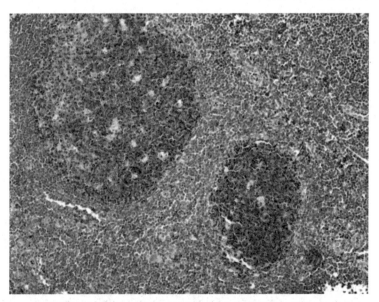

11. B cell responses are generated in germinal centres. These are illustrated as the discrete dark structures in this section of a tonsil.

germinal centre the B cells therefore undergo carefully coordinated rounds of proliferation.

The result of this is a surge in antibody-secreting B cells which eventually leave the lymph node and can be detected in the blood a week or so after an infection, accompanied by a rapid rise in antiviral antibodies. It is worth noting that not all antibodies directed against viral proteins are equal. Antibodies directed against the viral envelope proteins, which direct the attachment and infection of virus to host cells, are typically of the most protective value—although they are not always successful in neutralizing the target. If the virus is bound and recognized by the immune system in alternative ways (e.g. via complement) this may also provide some protection. Antibodies which bind a virus and prevent it infecting further cells are called *neutralizing antibodies*. Producing high levels of neutralizing antibodies is the goal of many vaccine strategies as this can provide complete protection against infection—a so-called *sterilizing immunity*.

The initial innate response and accompanying interferons, followed by rapidly emerging cellular (T cell) and humoral (B cell/antibody) immunity should reduce the number of productively infected cells and the spread of the virus between cells. This reduction in virus replication is important in the evolution of immunity since it means a reduced level of antigen and innate triggering. Here the B cell response and the T cell response diverge somewhat. B cells continue to mature and generate antibodies, and typically—after infection—these antibodies can be detected in the circulation for the rest of that person's life. Such antibodies are produced by B cells which have migrated to the bone marrow and actively secreted antibodies, having now become a specialized cell known as a *plasma cell*. T cells in contrast, are in the main much more short-lived. The response, as mentioned, expands very rapidly and *effector* CD8+ T cells reach very high numbers in the blood and tissues. In the absence of further stimulation, however, these cells die quickly and the population sharply contracts. This dynamic expansion and contraction makes sense in limiting the exposure of the body to very dangerous killer cells, which always have the potential to cause excessive tissue damage (i.e. *immunopathology*). However, this population is not lost altogether, persisting long-term as an immunological memory.

Laying down immunological memory

Immunological memory is considered the hallmark of adaptive immunity. It is on one level very simple—in fact it goes back to the definition of immunity in Chapter 1: immunological memory protects against a second exposure to the same infection. A person can be protected from a potentially fatal infection if the body has an immunological memory of the antigen. Such memory responses broadly work because the protective mediators (T cells, B cells, antibodies) are present in higher *quantities* and also possess appropriate *qualities* to fight a infection previously encountered infection. This combination of quantity and quality of these mediator cells means they can respond very quickly, leading to an absolute protection against infection, or at least a very rapid control and clearance of the infection before it has had time to establish itself or cause symptoms.

One of the most famous examples of memory induced by natural infection is that of an isolated Atlantic community in the Faroe Islands, who had been exposed to new infections only intermittently, through the arrival of seafarers. In 1846, the Danish physician Peter Panum went to the Faroes to investigate an outbreak of the measles virus—this virus has a very high attack rate in previously unexposed populations, with a high mortality rate in vulnerable groups (it killed one in five young children in an outbreak on the Pacific island of Rotuma in 1911). Panum noted that while the attack rate was indeed very high, a subset of individuals remained apparently uninfected—this was a group of elderly islanders who had been exposed to and survived a previous epidemic in 1781.

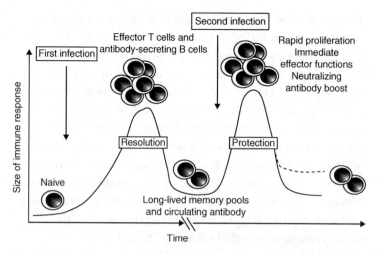

12. After the effector phase, the large pools of B and T cells contract and memory is established. Upon re-encounter with the same infection these will re-expand more rapidly and also can reach higher levels in the bloodstream (termed *boosting*).

Thus protective immunological memory established in one century had lasted half way through the next. It is very easy to imagine how such devastating infectious diseases could shape the evolution of the immune system (see Figure 12).

What processes underlie such long-lived protection? This question has long been debated by immunologists and continues to drive much interest in the field of vaccine research. Fortunately for the latter, a full understanding of this process has not been required in developing effective vaccines—simply harnessing the body's natural response to infection is enough in many cases. However, for complex infections such as HIV, looking under the bonnet of the memory response, taking the engine apart, and redesigning it will likely be required (see Chapter 7 for further discussion).

The best-understood part of the memory response, and broadly the most effective, is the induction of B cells and a very potent antibody that last for decades. B cells can improve the quality (stickiness or *affinity*) of their antibody over time. They do this by further adjusting the sequence of the immunoglobulin genes they originally made during the first few days of infection (see Chapter 3). The B cell of course does not know how to improve its antibody but takes the approach of an enthusiastic experimenter and attempts all available options in the hope of finding an antibody which works better. This process is controlled by a gene uniquely used by B cells—activation-induced cytosine deaminase (AID)—which deliberately mutates the relevant region of its immunoglobulin. AID works on an existing B cell response and helps improve the quality (affinity or stickiness) of the memory response (so called *affinity maturation*).

Memory antibody responses are also dominated by very active *IgG* antibodies that have a special additional quality which is that they cross the placenta. This is in contrast to the first antibodies that are made which are of *IgM* type (IgM antibodies are a good marker of there being an acute infection and are used for clinical diagnosis). One important consequence of this induction of strong IgG antibodies is that a mother's memory response can protect her unborn child against infection in utero. Beyond that it also is sufficiently long-lasting to continue to protect the newborn child. The level of transferred antibody drops in the baby over the first few months of life, but it serves to protect the baby effectively during his or her most vulnerable period. This added (perhaps *most* important) benefit happens naturally but could also be exploited further. For example, one interesting approach to vaccination against the virus Respiratory Syncitial Virus (RSV) currently being tested is to vaccinate pregnant women. This common disease is most severe in very young children and boosting maternal antibody levels is potentially a simple way of ensuring the youngest babies have sufficient protection at the time of greatest risk.

The B cell memory pool is organized in two parts—a set of *sleeper* memory cells, which reside in lymph nodes; and plasma cells, the highly differentiated set of B cells known as plasma cells (discussed earlier) which return to the bone marrow and are effectively antibody factories. This combination provides a balance within the immune system such that antibody-mediated protection can be sustained. Circulating specific antibodies provides immediate protection in neutralizing pathogens, and in some cases it is possible to infer the likelihood of successful protection by measuring the level of antibodies in the bloodstream (e.g. this test is done after vaccination against HBV to ensure a response has been made). The levels of these antibodies do however tend to wane over time after vaccination, and longer-term protection can be maintained by activation of the pool of memory B cells, which upon re-encountering the virus will rapidly proliferate and generate further antibody-secreting cells and high antibody levels. This means that even decades after an exposure, the system is primed to rapidly secrete further antibodies and provide effective protection.

T cell memory and its distribution

T cell memory is somewhat more complex since there is no simple marker like the antibody level equating to *protective immunity*. Nevertheless, we do understand the types of memory T cell that are induced and their likely roles in host defence, which is roughly parallel to those seen in B cells (this is true for both killer CD8+ and helper CD4+ T cells) (see Figure 13). Thus one set of T cells becomes the sleeper set, not actively functional but ready to respond in the case of re-exposure to the infection. These are located within lymph nodes and the spleen—ideal sites to re-encounter antigens if they are presented on an antigen-presenting cell (e.g. in the priming phase).

A second set of T cells has a more active lifestyle, homing in on peripheral tissues (such as the liver, gut, lung, etc.) and maintaining some elements of *effector functions* (killing capacity for CD8+ T cells and immediate secretion of specific cytokines).

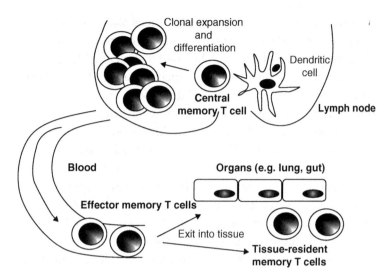

13. Central memory T cells are found enriched in lymph nodes. Effector memory cells are found in the bloodstream and enriched in peripheral organs. A further set of T cell memory cells are found resident in tissues.

These latter cells look in many ways like acute effector cells and have been termed *effector* memory in contrast with the sleeper cells found in lymph nodes which are termed *central* memory. Central memory cells, in response to an antigen previously encountered, will proliferate and acquire effector functions, homing in on tissues again, so the two populations are not independent of each other. In certain low-level chronic infections, such as CMV, the virus is never fully cleared, so there is a continuous activation of the memory pool and accompanying proliferation of these cells. The net result is that very large populations of effector memory CD8+ T cells can gradually accumulate in response to a single peptide, sometimes taking up about a third of the entire T cell memory population in the bloodstream (a process described as *memory inflation*).

In addition to these localization differences, there are other ways the T cell memory population can diversify, helping to tune the immune response against specific threats. For example, it has recently emerged that some populations of memory T cells found in tissues appear to have migrated there permanently—so-called *resident* memory cells. These may have a specific role in very early responses to infection in tissue, before it is fully established. Certainly overall, T cells play a distinct role in tissue defence and, unlike B cells which can act remotely via secreted antibodies, their immediate presence and local effector functions are required to protect the barrier surface.

Other T cells have developed a lifestyle focused on the germinal centre. T cell assistance in the germinal centre reaction is crucial in generating long-lived B cell memory. Vaccinologists have learned to harness this by attaching the target of interest to a specific protein which in turn attracts and activates these helper cells—a so-called *conjugate* vaccine. The newer vaccines against the pneumococcus (*Streptococcus pneumoniae*, the major cause of pneumonia in children and the elderly) are very effective and based on this principle. Further subtypes of T cell also can develop during such responses which have specialized properties. These include Type 2 cells, which are involved in defence against worms and also in allergy; and Type 17 cells, involved in defence against bacteria and yeasts. These will be dealt with in Chapters 5 and 6.

Harnessing B and T cell memories for immune protection

Having explored the mechanics of memory formation, let us consider how this has been harnessed in current vaccines and how this understanding may inform future vaccine development. The classic vaccines are called *live attenuated* vaccines, which are typically viruses that have been grown in tissue culture and have become less *virulent* (i.e. less able to cause disease) in the process. Vaccinia, the first vaccine used by Edward Jenner for protection against smallpox, is a related virus to smallpox but found as an infection in cows—it infects humans but causes a much milder and more limited disease. Since such vaccines are based upon viruses, they induce a response which mirrors that of a real infection, starting with recognition of innate triggers, antigen presentation, and induction of B and T cell responses to the presented antigens, followed by long-term memory formation. Providing the antigens are the same or largely shared between the vaccine and the real pathogen, a broad and protective response can be induced. This really is the ideal setting, as long-lived effective immunity can be readily generated—it may even be that since the pathogen is *live*, it may persist at tiny levels in specific niches, sufficient to keep subtly boosting the immune response in the long term. Such vaccines have provided protection against infections such as measles, influenza, and polio to countless populations, and vaccination has led to the eradication of smallpox (see Figure 14).

Another simple approach is to use a protein antigen. For example, this works well in inducing responses against the toxin in *Clostridium tetani*—an organism found in the soil which can

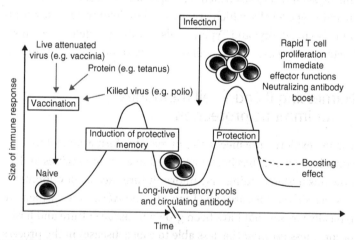

14. This figure shows the same process as described for memory following infection—only in this case it is induced by a vaccine. The same induction of memory T and B cells occurs, and these exert the same protective effects upon encountering the true infection.

infect wounds, leading to tetanus. Antibodies against the bacteria are not needed, simply the neutralization of the dangerous toxin, which is a protein. Administration of tetanus *toxoid*, where the protein toxin is inactivated by a simple treatment and made harmless, is followed by the induction of effective antibodies—and these block the activity of this highly potent toxin. A similar vaccine approach works against the toxin *Corynebacterium diphtheriae* (the bacterium which causes diphtheria). Both vaccines were developed in the 1920s by Ramon and Descombey and have remained virtually unchanged for nearly a century, saving countless lives over that time.

Protein antigens are typically administered with an *adjuvant*—a substance which causes non-specific inflammation and so enhances immunity. One such commonly used adjuvant is alum (aluminium salts), which can activate various innate pathways, although perhaps in future specifically designed adjuvants may become available, taking advantage of our new knowledge about the pathways that are necessary for full priming of B and T cells. They also generally need boosting, as the protein can be readily cleared, and repeated exposure is needed to drive the B cells through the germinal centre reactions required for expansion, affinity maturation, and class switching. Also such vaccines typically require boosting at a later interval, as the levels of antibodies tend to drop and further memory pools and plasma cells are required to sustain this. However, despite these limitations, protein-based vaccines to induce antibodies are hugely effective. Similar progress has been made using inactivated versions of whole viruses—for example, Louis Pasteur's rabies vaccine, which protects completely against a disease which is otherwise universally fatal.

Vaccines against bacteria such as Mtb (see Chapters 2 and 3), which live inside the cell and so would not be affected by antibodies or B cells, are much harder to develop—but there are several major targets. The oldest of these vaccines—and the only one licensed—is BCG, which is a live attenuated form of Mtb, which infects about two billion people globally. BCG (Bacille Calmette–Guérin), which was developed at the Pasteur Institute, has lost significant portions of its genome and is consequently highly *attenuated*. This vaccine has been trialled in many countries and can provide effective protection for children—a group in whom the disease can be very severe. However, its efficacy in adults is much less clear. Mtb sets up an intracellular infection just like viruses, so T cell-mediated immunity is important in its clearance. However, unlike antibodies, where it is possible to assign a protective function to a certain level of specific antibodies in the blood, defining what would be a protective level of immunity against Mtb and which of the many proteins it should possess as the best target is not straightforward. The task is made somewhat harder as Mtb shares antigens with harmless mycobacteria, which we are all exposed to, and which might influence the response to BCG (or newer vaccines) in later life.

One utility of immunological memory that has been harnessed for human benefit is the ability to transfer immunity from one person to another—so-called *passive immunity*. This was alluded to in the context of the transmission of antibodies from mother to child, where it happens naturally, but antibodies can be purified or concentrated for clinical use. One example of such treatment is to replace missing memory in individuals who lack the capacity to induce their own immunoglobulins. Simply transferring immunoglobulins of broad specificities at regular intervals can protect these individuals against serious infections. Such passive immunization has been used by doctors for many years in specific cases—for example, potent antisera can be used to protect individuals who are not immune but have been exposed to HBV, chickenpox (in cases where they are immunosuppressed or pregnant), or rabies. It can also be used after a snake bite to neutralize venom. The development of highly targeted monoclonal antibodies of a single specificity has huge potential in this area (see also Chapter 7).

The idea of memory in this context has long fascinated immunologists and neuroscientists alike. In both cases the development of a long-lived 'imprint' of an event is through a complex, multi-cellular system where the information is not stored or retrieved at a single site. Even if it is possible to identify lymphocytes we label as 'memory', they only act as part of a much larger team. In both cases, an element of rehearsal serves to fix the memory in the system—repetitive antigen stimulation or long-lived infections have an enormous impact in moulding the memory state. In both cases it even appears that false memories can be created—this is a natural by-product of cross-reactivity in the immune system. The consequences of such false memory in the shape of auto-immunity is dealt with in Chapter 6. Developing memories in advance, or 'getting your retaliation in first' to quote a British Lions rugby coach, through vaccines, has saved countless lives since the time of Jenner, and has the potential to save many more in the face of emerging infectious threats.

Chapter 5
Too little immunity: immunological failure

The immune system functions so well that most of the time we do not notice it is actually working at all. However, it is continuously active, preventing severe infection from the micro-organisms which colonize our skin and our gut, and suppressing the chronic virus infections most of us picked up as infants. In certain individuals, or under certain conditions, the immune response may, however, fail and this can lead to severe disease, the exact disease depending on the precise mechanism of failure. In this chapter we will examine how such failures may occur—specifically through genetic changes and through HIV infection—and also what we may learn from them about the working of the normal immune system.

Redundancy, polymorphisms, and knockouts

The immune system is a complex machine with multiple parts. In an ideal situation, every part functions perfectly, with induction of appropriate levels of immunity against commensal bacteria (i.e. not too much) and robust defence against infectious threats (i.e. just enough). If certain aspects fail, a number of outcomes are possible—in the same way as failing parts of a car have different impacts. One quite reasonable outcome is that nothing at all happens. For such a critical system there is apparently some inbuilt redundancy. For example, humans have multiple forms of interferon alpha, all of which do more or less the same job (i.e. protect cells against virus infection). One of the critical entry receptors for HIV is a molecule called CCR5, which is a chemokine receptor giving T cells information about where to traffic. Although the molecule is widespread, inherited deficiency of CCR5 has minimal impact on the health of the host, although as we will discuss later it has a huge impact on HIV infection. Losing some molecules is perhaps analogous to losing the spare tyre—not noticeable as long as the other four tyres are okay.

Other genetic defects have an enormous impact. Loss of the so-called *common gamma chain*, which is critical to the signalling of a number of molecules essential for lymphocyte growth and survival, leads to the development of severe combined immunodeficiency. Under these conditions most lymphocyte subsets simply fail to develop normally and the affected host is highly immunosuppressed. Another example was discussed in Chapter 1, where the thymus fails to develop in DiGeorge's syndrome, leading to a catastrophic failure of T cell immunity. This sort of defect is comparable to a large hole in the petrol tank—the car simply cannot run even if the rest of the machinery is intact.

There are a large number of other defects in the immune system—or subtle differences between people (genetic polymorphisms)—that have a more specific effect on immune defence. Loss of particular innate signalling genes can yield susceptibility to a narrow range of infections (such as rare viral infections of the brain). Mutations in a specific set of interferon genes (interferon lambda 3 and 4) can affect the rate of clearance of HCV and also the response to therapy—but apparently little else. They are perhaps, to continue the car analogy, more like losing a nearside mirror—most of the time this might not be noticeable but there will be a specific blind spot affecting particular manoeuvres. These specific relationships are of particular interest as they can

57

tell us a lot about the bespoke requirements needed to protect against individual infectious threats, and how the immune system has evolved to deal with them.

Considering the differences between us that might influence the quality of immune responses (small differences known as genetic *polymorphisms*), the most important area of the human genome is the MHC, responsible for what is known as *tissue type* or HLA-type (see Figure 15). As discussed in Chapter 3, these molecules are responsible for presenting peptide fragments derived from pathogens to TCRs on T cells. Only those parts of a virus where the peptides can be bound into the groove of the MHC molecule are actually visible to the cellular immune system—T cells are more or less blind to the other parts. It is as if the MHC molecules need to reveal the information given by the virus, the rest being hidden.

The MHC is the most diverse part of the human genome—it has undergone intense selection over time, leading to a huge diversity

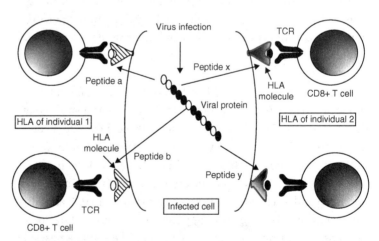

15. Individual 1 has a set of HLA molecules that, upon infection with a virus, may present peptides a and b; while individual 2 will present peptides x and y. In effect, their immune systems are 'seeing' the same virus quite differently.

of MHC molecules in the human population. Thus individuals' MHC molecules vary quite widely in terms of the peptides they select for presentation—and this can make a very big difference to the immune response which is made. In other words, although two individuals may be infected at the same time with exactly the same virus, the peptides presented to their T cells may be entirely different between the two people. In some situations this might make no difference—all T cell responses might be equally good. In others, however, the exact choice of peptide can be critical. This is particularly the case in chronic virus infections such as HIV and HCV. Here, peptide choice can be crucial. Certain MHC molecules focus the immune response on areas of the virus which are more effective targets, thus giving the T cells a relative advantage. Those born with such favourable genetics have a better outcome following infection (see HIV, discussed later in this chapter). Similarly, there are unfavourable MHC types which appear to direct a less effective immune response either because of high variability in the viral peptide targets or even through lack of such targets.

The ability to respond to a range of peptides is clearly crucial for an individual to give them the best chance of finding a suitable target on a virus. Across a population it is also an advantage to have a diversity of such choice so that viruses cannot adapt to escape responses generally. There are data to suggest that mate choice (including in humans) can be driven by olfactory signals derived from such MHC molecules—such that those with divergent MHC types are chosen, hence maximizing the number of different MHC molecules available to the offspring. Not all animals are so lucky—in chicken colonies, where there is very limited MHC choice, viruses such as Marek's disease have succeeded in adapting to the host immunity in order to enhance their infection. In humans, even though the range of MHCs remains very wide, it is still observed that viruses such as HIV may adapt over time across a population level to evade recognition by MHCs and thus T cells. MHC molecules are in this way said to leave their 'footprints' on the virus—but similarly through such intensive selection, viruses have left their footprints on the MHC too.

The MHC and the peptides it presents are so central to immune responses that MHC (or HLA) type is linked to a wide range of diseases (including auto-immunity, as will be seen in Chapter 6). However, it is not the only example where natural variation in human genetics can lead to weaker or stronger immune responses, even if the range is narrower. An important example is also seen in HCV infection, where it was identified that natural variation around the interferon lambda region was strongly linked to outcome of infection. In the case of infection with this virus, some individuals are able to clear infection spontaneously as a result of an effective immune response. With a particular mutation in the interferon lambda region this rate was increased around four to fivefold, and also increased the chance of successful clearance following treatment.

Interferon lambdas are a subset of interferons which share many of the same anti-infective properties as interferon alpha and beta already described, but which have a more limited tissue range—particularly working in tissues such as the liver and lung. The protective gene type is actually almost universal in some populations, so there may have been some selective force driving this—although it is to date unclear whether it impacts on any other infection. This is perhaps an example of a 'wing mirror' gene—critical for optimal function of the immune system but only in rather specific circumstances.

Inborn errors of the immune system

Some genetic changes lead to specific loss of a gene—a 'knockout'. These can also have rather pinpoint effects on the human immune system (see Figure 16). Although rare, such mutations can uncover a critical role for a specific pathway in control of certain

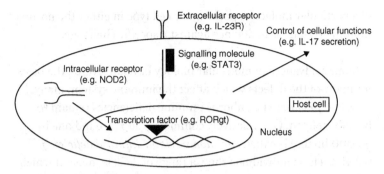

16. Defects in host defence can occur through mutations in cell surface receptors, signalling molecules, transcription factors, or effector molecules. Recognition molecules such as TLRs and NOD2 can impact on early events in immune activation.

infections. One example here would be loss of the Type 17 pathway, revealing a critical role for the pathway for the control of fungal infections. Individuals carrying mutations that affect this pathway, such as mutations in the extracellular receptor IL-23R, the signalling molecule STAT3, the master regulator transcription factor RORgt (which controls the cells using the Type 17 pathway), or in genes controlling cellular functions such as IL-17 secretion, suffer repeated and persistent fungal infections. This does not mean that the Type 17 pathway is only involved in fungal defence—experiments show that it is clearly involved in defending against bacteria as well—but it does indicate that its role in fungal defence is unique and cannot be performed by any other pathway.

Such human genetic data linked to human immune responses are very valuable but also very rare. In the last decades, enormous advances have been made by analysis of mouse models where specific defects have been engineered. The mouse immune system has been very well studied and many methods exist to examine the response to infection, tumours, and other diseases. To address the question of the role of a specific molecule it is now possible to introduce a genetic defect in a precisely targeted way into the mouse. This is a particularly powerful technique to define the role of a particular molecule, pathway, or cell type in either the normal immune system or in defence against a specific challenge.

Although advances in molecular biology have uncovered the basis for many of the defects which affect the immune system, many so-called *primary* (i.e. inborn) immune deficiencies remain to be fully defined. One relatively common group (around one in 50,000 births) is called *common variable immunodeficiency* (CVID). These individuals show a range of defects, most of which affect the ability to make effective antibody responses. Since the pathway to making an antibody is a long one, involving B cells and T cells cooperating around an antigen, a number of different defects affecting cell function and survival can lead to the same result. For those affected, they are susceptible to infection—most obviously, bacterial infections of the lungs. Repeated infections that are poorly controlled can lead to destructive lung damage (*bronchiectasis*), which in itself can badly impact on the normal immune defence system.

This clinical presentation does point to the critical role of antibodies in keeping control over the very common organisms that we all harbour such as *Streptococcus pneumoniae*. Other sites such as the gut, urinary tract, and eyes can also be affected—sites which can come into contact with bacteria regularly or continuously. Additionally, the immune dysregulation can be associated with auto-immune phenomena, indicating how finely balanced the system is under normal conditions. Fortunately, once it is diagnosed (which is not always straightforward, as it may take time to fully declare itself), treatment with transfusions of immunoglobulins from healthy donors can provide protection against the infectious complications of this disease. Since immunoglobulin levels decline with a half life of around three weeks, in the absence of a genetic cure, this therapy is regular and lifelong. It may be that with better molecular definition of the underlying causes in each case, alternative approaches to repair of the specific defects could be developed.

Malnutrition and immunodeficiency

At a global level, and throughout human history, an important cause of immunodeficiency is malnutrition. This can take a number of forms, including loss of specific micronutrients, such as vitamins and minerals, as well as protein-calorie malnutrition, which may well coexist. The exact impact of such malnutrition is variable depending on the function of the molecule—for example Vitamin D is involved in the development of regulatory T cells, while the Vitamin A pathway is involved in signals driving mucosal defence. T cells possess receptors for hormones involved in starvation. It has been shown that leptin, an important satiety hormone (i.e. one that suppresses appetite) can act not only on the brain but also to inhibit T cell function, providing a possible link between starvation (where leptin levels are high) and immune dysfunction. This is a complex area, where multiple different effects may overlap—worm infections, which are prevalent globally, can directly influence the immune system (see Chapter 6), as well as impacting on nutritional status and leading to iron loss, all of which could influence the response to infections with other micro-organisms.

HIV and Acquired Immunodeficiency Syndrome (AIDS)

How do pathogens exploit a normal immune system? One approach is to disable it, and this method is used by most viruses in order to create a specific niche or window of time in which to replicate. One virus above all has developed a strategy to exploit the immune system and turn it to its own advantage to devastating effect. HIV-1 (and its less prevalent relation HIV-2, found mainly in West Africa) is related to viruses found in many strains of African primates, including chimpanzees. It crossed over into human populations likely in the mid part of the 20th century. Like many viruses that cross species, it causes quite a different disease in each new host. Thus HIV relatives (so-called Simian Immunodeficiency Viruses or SIVs) can be carried in certain monkey species relatively harmlessly. This is probably a process of co-evolution, whereby the virus has adapted to the host to limit pathology and additionally the host populations have evolved to survive the infections. However, upon crossing species, the rules of engagement are rewritten and HIV-1 not only evades the human immune system but it also dismantles it (see Figure 17).

The first reason that HIV-1 is devastating to the immune system is because of the cell it targets for infection. HIV-1 uses two molecules in order to gain access to cells—CD4 and a chemokine receptor, typically CCR5. CD4 is the major molecule marking out T helper cells—it is the co-receptor for the MHC Class II molecules used for recognition by the T cell receptor. CCR5 is a receptor which allows the T cells to home in on sites of infection or inflammation, following cues laid down by other cells in the form of chemokine trails. Thus by using such receptors the virus is able to target T helper cells, particularly cells which have been recently activated. Infection of such cells can lead to a range of outcomes, none of which are good for the host. The cell may

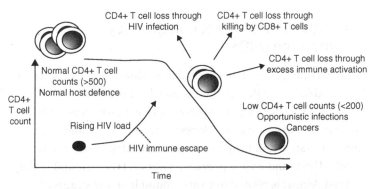

17. CD4+ T cells are normally present at levels greater than 500 cells per microlitre of blood, but they fall as HIV infection progresses, which in turn is associated with rising viral load. Below 200 cells per microlitre the host is at high risk of opportunistic infections.

become productively infected and generate more viruses. It may be recognized by the immune response and destroyed by CD8+ T cells. Or the virus may integrate and lay down a latent form for later reactivation.

The development of latency is a specific feature of the group of viruses to which HIV belongs—so-called retroviruses. These viruses are so-called as they are based as RNA, but can copy themselves back into DNA using a specific enzyme called *reverse transcriptase*. This DNA form of the virus is stable and is the template used to copy further versions of the virus genome and all the proteins required for virus function. It can be integrated into the host genome using a specific *integrase* enzyme which inserts the viral copy in among the host genetic material. If the virus is active, viral proteins will be generated and the cell will become a target for CD8+ T cells. However, if it is quiescent it will be invisible to the immune system and can persist as long as the cell (or its progeny) survives. This feature alone makes the virus very difficult to eliminate completely.

The infection of CD4+ T cells on its own would be a significant insult to the immune system if it resulted in a substantial loss of such cells—but if it were short-lived, it is likely such cells would recover rapidly. The fundamental problem with HIV is its ability to set up persistent infection, and thus the impact on the immune system is prolonged and extensive. How does HIV achieve this? One feature has already been mentioned—the development of a latent pool. However, while this represents real issues in terms of elimination in the long run, the persistence which occurs is associated with very high levels of virus in the bloodstream—thus active replication in the face of host immunity. One answer to this can be found by analysing the evolution of the virus within a host and observing the rapid adaptation to an individual host. The copying mechanism of HIV by reverse transcriptase has an interesting defect which means that the new copies are not 'proofread'. Thus each new copy of the virus contains at least one mutation. Given that there are trillions of copies of the virus generated daily and each contains around 10,000 base pairs in its genome, this means that every possible mutation it can make is potentially available to the virus. This huge pool of variants provides a rich resource for Darwinian selection, and this is exactly what is observed in the face of attack from B and T cells.

The antibody targets for HIV lie in the viral envelope—a difficult target since it is heavily *glycosylated* (i.e. coated in sugar molecules)—the molecules acting as a shield. Some of the most important and vulnerable areas are also hidden deeply and only open up on engagement with the cell to allow entry. Nevertheless, effective antibodies can be generated against HIV which should be able to neutralize and block infection by a given virus. However, single mutations in the virus genome can readily protect the virus against such antibodies and the development of such mutations in the envelope is exactly what is observed throughout infection. In other words, the immune system is able to control effectively any given virus strain through generation of antibodies, but the virus is able to remain one step ahead by generating new strains—the mutations often appearing to come at little cost to the virus.

So-called *broadly neutralizing antibodies* (bNABs), in other words, antibodies which could neutralize a very wide range of HIV mutants and so protect against infection, are a holy grail for HIV research. Indeed, these antibodies do develop after infection, but they take a long time to generate. If these could be generated using a simple vaccine approach, for example by focusing the immune response on the specific target from the start, this would be a huge breakthrough for the field.

The virus is, however, also under attack from the CD8+ T cell response and here additionally the ability to generate mutations gives the virus an advantage. Certain MHC types such as HLA-B27 and HLA-B57 are associated with better outcomes following HIV infection. A very rare group of patients who carry HIV are able to suppress it down to extremely low levels without suffering from progressive loss of CD4+ T cells. These so-called *elite controllers* are highly enriched for certain HLA types such as HLA-B27 and HLA-B57 (although other factors are also involved). These molecules bind peptides in the virus Gag protein, a molecule used to package the viral genome within the virus. Gag is relatively constrained in its ability to mutate compared to the viral envelope, and thus if the virus is forced to mutate to evade recognition by T cells, there may be a consequence for its Gag protein in terms of fitness. That is, every mutation that is made could subtly impact on the way that the protein functions, and so could impair the ability of the virus to replicate—a so-called *fitness cost*.

One way for the virus to manage this balancing act is to make multiple mutations to find a way of evading recognition while limiting the fitness cost. In such elite controllers therefore the virus is effectively pinned into a corner where it has a much more limited range of options to explore in terms of mutants and has already some compromise to its fitness. However, such outcomes are relatively rare. For the average person infected with HIV, the virus is able to mutate its T cell epitopes to escape the CD8+ T cell response and replicate effectively.

There are other factors which serve to limit the impact of the antiviral response and allow HIV not only to persist but to replicate to high levels. One is a specific down-regulation of the antiviral immune response referred to as exhaustion. This process occurs under settings where an immune response is very prolonged and is accompanied by up-regulation of off switches or checkpoints. The most well-known of these is *PD-1* (programmed death 1) which is able to limit T cell functions when it engages with its target, PD-1 ligand. This process is certainly active during prolonged HIV infection, and expression of a range of checkpoint molecules associated with the exhausted phenotype is linked to failure to control the virus. In the mouse model of LCMV (Lymphocytic Choriomeningitis Virus), where a similar process occurs during persistent infection, blockade of PD-1 can rejuvenate the T cell response and is associated with virus control. Such approaches are a potential avenue in infectious disease but have been much more influential in cancer therapies. Ultimately 'exhausted' T cell populations may simply be lost—or deleted. In HIV, it is not clear to what extent the T cell responses are truly exhausted, but any regulation of the immune response which limits the ability of CD8+ T cells to eliminate productively infected targets subtly shifts the balance of power in favour of the pathogen within the cell.

Although escape and exhaustion play an important role in allowing HIV to persist, this does not fully explain the massive loss of CD4+ T cells seen in HIV. Only a relatively small fraction of CD4+ T cells may be infected with the virus, but the impact is seen across the entire population. One explanation for this amplified effect is the development of *immune activation*: T cells which have been activated express certain surface markers such as HLA Class II molecules, allowing them to be tracked. The magnitude of general immune activation in HIV has long been found to indicate a worse outcome. It is likely that activated immune cells undergo more rapid turnover and death, and they are also more susceptible to HIV infection.

One of the prevailing theories for why immune activation may occur is that early in infection there is substantial infection of the CD4+ T cells in the gut. Normally these cells play an important role in barrier defence, and loss of such a barrier may lead to very low-grade transit of bacteria from the gut into the bloodstream (so-called *bacterial translocation*). Although this is insufficient to cause major infection, it is sufficient to activate the innate sensors in the immune system and trigger T cell activation. The long-term consequences of very early T cell infection in the gut may therefore be via this very indirect mechanism, although other innate responses to the virus itself may also contribute. Of relevance to this argument, the monkey strains which harbour

SIV without any harm (such as Sooty Mangabeys) show very low levels of such immune activation, despite carrying high levels of virus.

HIV infection therefore leads to loss of CD4+ T cells through direct infection, immune-mediated killing, indirect effects of immune activation, and likely many other mechanisms. HIV also can infect macrophages in tissues (which express low levels of CD4) and dendritic cells, and there are indirect effects leading to depletion of other cell types such as MAIT cells. However, of all of these the CD4+ T cell count in the blood is the best measure for the progression of the infection and the patient's risk of disease. The lower this drops, the greater the susceptibility to a range of pathogens, many of which are so-called *opportunistic*.

Even healthy persons are susceptible to TB infection, but the requirement for a fully intact cellular immune response to provide defence against TB means that, even relatively early on, the risk of disease is markedly increased. In contrast, there are a number of related mycobacterial infections which are never seen in a healthy immune system but become increasingly prevalent at low CD4+ T cell counts. At such low counts (<200 cells per cubic millimetre, where a normal count is >500) the patients are susceptible to a wide range of opportunistic infections including intracellular protozoan parasites such as *Toxoplasma gondii* (causing brain lesions), gut pathogens (e.g. *Cryptosporidium* species causing diarrhoea), yeasts, and fungi (e.g. *Pneumocystis jirovecii* causing pneumonia), and viruses such as the JC virus which can cause devastating destruction of brain tissue. These are all organisms which will be dealt with readily by a healthy immune system, but clearly these severe illnesses show the ongoing role of CD4+ T cells in coordinating that system.

One further disease category seen in such patients with acquired immunodeficiency is that of cancer. Two of the major cancers seen, Kaposi's sarcoma and B cell lymphomas, are driven by different viruses (HHV-8 and Epstein–Barr Virus or EBV, respectively). These viruses are both from the same group and are normally hard to eliminate in healthy individuals (EBV is a very common infection), but they are usually well controlled and cause little harm long-term. Uncontrolled replication is linked to the transformation of normal cells into cancer cells—thus such virally driven cancers are further examples of the central role of CD4+ T cells in controlling normal host defence against common antigens.

HIV is a devastating infection and—for the reasons described in this chapter—we still lack an effective vaccine. However, drug treatments are very effective at suppressing virus replication and halting the progression of the disease. Restoration of CD4+ T cell counts is, largely, associated with recovery of immune function and protection against opportunistic infections and cancers. Nevertheless, treatment is only suppressive—thus therapy must be taken lifelong with only one reported case of a person attaining a complete cure. This is one individual who has received a bone marrow transplant to treat a blood cancer, and in this transplant the marrow was from a donor who had a mutation in the CCR5 molecule. This mutation is relatively common and can influence the natural infection rate—if the person has two copies of the mutant gene this renders them highly resistant to HIV. The recipient of the transplant was able to effectively inherit this status with the donated marrow and subsequently has remained free of virus without further treatment. Unfortunately, so far, this individual remains the only example of such a cure.

This is a somewhat unusual and drastic therapy, but various attempts are being made to eliminate HIV from its long-term reservoirs in the body and provide an effective cure. As described earlier, the ability to lay down a latent pool gives the virus an enormous advantage over the host—the immune system is not able to visualize and respond to cells where the virus is not replicating, and drugs are equally inactive. One approach is to activate the virus using a range of approaches and then destroy the cells which have revealed their virus before they go on to spread it further. This is a complex area, since the actual site of the cells where the reservoir is located, their status, and the means to fully eliminate them are all poorly defined. As such, for the time being the main thrust must be to get as many people who need therapy onto an effective treatment and to stop the spread of infection by means of education and appropriate interventions (including pre-exposure treatment programmes). In the meantime, the search for an effective HIV vaccine continues.

Chapter 6
Too much immunity: auto-immunity and allergic diseases

Much of the emphasis so far in this book has been on providing defence against micro-organisms, and this is the major driving force for the evolution of the immune system. This is clear from the severe disease syndromes that occur when the immune system is deficient (seen Chapter 5). However, given the capacity to cause tissue damage and inflammation, every immune response must be appropriately and specifically tuned. Failure to tune in appropriately leads to a range of immunologically driven diseases that, given the general improvements in health status and many major infections in Western populations, have taken on increasing significance. In this chapter we will address how the immune system acts to turn off unwanted responses, and what goes wrong when this fails. This includes looking not only at classical auto-immune diseases but also at other diseases where there is excessive inflammation. It also includes consideration of allergic diseases, where there is an exaggerated response to harmless antigens, dominated by a particular style of immunity.

Tolerance in the thymus

To understand how auto-immune diseases occur it is important to review how the immune system takes steps to avoid this—by so-called *immune tolerance*. The rules are somewhat different for T and B cells, but since CD4+ T cells are crucial for the development of most long-lived antibody responses, if the T cells are well controlled then the B cell compartment will follow. T cells are educated primarily in the thymus, so this is the most critical site where self-tolerance is learned.

One puzzle for T cells is how to ensure the TCRs that are generated are of any use. Since the T cell puts the TCR together at random and the recognition of an antigen is completely dependent on the MHC molecules present in that individual, it is likely that many TCRs are of no value in an immune response. This is not the case for B cells, where the antigen could be very broad—a protein, a sugar molecule, a lipid (fat), or even a chemical. The problem is solved by providing some early education for the T cells in the thymus. Two essential processes take place in the thymus—so-called *positive* and *negative* selection (see Figure 18). Positive selection is a process to ensure that the repertoire has some ability to recognize

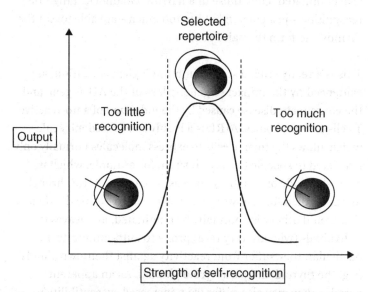

18. The T cell (CD4+ or CD8+) will encounter self-antigens as it develops in the thymus. Those T cells where such interactions are too strong or too weak are eliminated (i.e. central tolerance).

self-MHC—in other words, the particular suite of MHC molecules present in that person.

Upon entry into the thymus as a very early and immature cell, the T cells start to arrange their T cell receptors. As we discussed in Chapter 3, there is a huge range available; what is required are receptors which are able to engage with the person's own MHC molecules but not react against self. This is an interesting balancing act as no pathogens are available in the thymus of a developing foetus or newborn child on which to base this choice of self versus non-self. The way the immune system solves this problem is to present a wide range of self-peptides in the thymus through the activity of a specific gene called *AIRE*. This allows the cells in the thymus to make proteins normally made only in very specialized cells in the body (e.g. from the pancreas or brain) and then eliminate T cells which react against these. Similarly, T cells which completely fail to engage with the self-MHC are also eliminated. Only those in a narrow 'Goldilocks range' of recognition—just enough but not too much—are able to exit the thymus and form the naive pool.

This is a really crucial step in immunological education, as evidenced by the impact of genetic loss of the AIRE gene and the consequent disease caused by the induction of auto-reactive T cells and antibodies. AIRE is a highly specialized molecule which allows the thymic cells to express molecules normally only restricted to specific tissues—insulin, for example, which is normally made only in the pancreas. The loss of AIRE through mutation therefore allows a range of T cells to escape the thymus that would otherwise normally be eliminated, and leaves the individuals (who are very rare) prone to auto-immunity. In particular, they suffer from reactivity against their own glands (e.g. the thyroid and parathyroid glands). As an apparent paradox they may also suffer from increased susceptibility to yeast infections—but this is due to antibodies fighting their own cytokine Interleukin 17. As we saw in Chapter 5, Interleukin 17 is crucial in defence against surface Candida infections, so this combination of auto-immunity and immunodeficiency is the result of the same process of lack of self-tolerance.

Peripheral tolerance

However, even if AIRE is fully functional, this process is still not sufficient to protect fully against auto-immunity, and a 'belt and braces' approach is taken by the immune system. Tolerance can be broken, for example, if a rogue T cell escapes the thymus without having been properly educated, or if there is very close mimicry between a pathogen and a self-protein. This may sound unlikely, but what is actually recognized by the T cell receptor is a short peptide, which is bound in the MHC groove and presents perhaps only two to three major amino acids that are recognized. Thus even if the peptides themselves differ between, say, a virus and a protein from the brain, by the time it has been bound and presented in the MHC, the overall shape recognized may overlap somewhat. The thymic system thus must be flexible enough to allow T cells to escape where such cross-reactivity may exist, otherwise the ability to respond to pathogens would be excessively limited. In other words, it is somewhat leaky—or the immune system needs to take a small risk in releasing T cells.

But if rogue (or potentially rogue) T cells are circulating in all of us, why do we not all succumb to auto-immunity? One possibility is just ignorance. If antigens are hidden away, and therefore not presented to the immune system on an antigen-presenting cell such as a dendritic cell (by the processes described in Chapter 3), the immune response will never be triggered. This phenomenon may account for lack of responsiveness to specific tissues such as the brain, which is protected by the blood–brain barrier, a physical barrier that largely excludes cells of the immune system from entering the brain. However, in experimental models it is still possible to induce auto-reactivity against the brain by vaccination with brain-derived proteins or peptides—such peripherally induced cells are able to cross into the brain and cause disease, so such a 'Maginot line'-style defence is not adequate for complete protection.

Tissues also protect themselves. Some possess mechanisms to down-regulate T cells—for example, they may express death receptors (Fas-ligand) which engage molecules on T cells to kill them. PD-1, which we discussed previously in the context of immune exhaustion, is also an important off-signal for T cells. Mice that lack PD-1 are highly prone to auto-immune disease. This is a very interesting example whereby viruses have essentially harnessed an off switch present in the immune system to down-regulate immune responses and allow them to persist. Another similar inhibitory molecule is called CTLA4. CTLA4 is expressed on T cells and binds the same molecules as an activatory receptor called CD28. CD28 triggering is very important in the initiation of immune responses—but CTLA4 can interfere with this and abrogate such reactivity. Mutations leading to loss of CTLA4 lead to severe auto-immune disease, with marked proliferation of lymphocytes. Interestingly, CTLA4 possesses a number of variants in the population and certain variants are strongly linked to auto-immune disease of the liver, thyroid, pancreas (causing diabetes mellitus), and gut. These variants can be posited to tune the immune reactivity of the host, and in combination with other similarly subtle defects can contribute to the development of clinical auto-immune syndromes.

As we learned in Chapter 5, rare inherited diseases can beautifully illustrate the importance of specific cells or pathways, and IPEX syndrome is one such example. Here there is loss of FOXP3, a molecule which is essential for the development of a set of T cells described as T regulatory cells or *Tregs*. Loss of Tregs is associated with severe auto-immunity and these cells clearly play an important role in maintenance of a healthy, steady state in all of us. Tregs can be derived via a number of routes, and have a range of specificities—but they are all able to act on other immune cells, notably other T cells, to inhibit their proliferation and many other functions. Some Tregs are actually derived from the thymus—rather than deleting auto-reactive cells the thymus actually turns them to good use by inducing a regulatory programme. These Tregs exit the thymus and can help to control auto-reactivity through the release of inhibitory cytokines such as Interleukin 10 and Tissue Growth Factor beta (TGFb). They also express high levels of the Interleukin 2 (IL-2) receptor CD25—a molecule used as an important surface marker for such cells. Interleukin 2 will be sensed by Tregs even at low levels and enhances their function—when auto-reactive T cells are activated IL-2 is made, and this can enhance Treg activity and limit auto-immune disease.

Because of the way T cells are sequentially selected in the thymus, if a self-reactive T cell is generated against a specific target, a Treg will be similarly generated to essentially keep an eye on it in the periphery. However, if needed, Tregs may also be induced in the periphery from otherwise standard T cells—these also develop through expression of FOXP3 and development of regulatory activity and upregulation of the IL-2 receptor. The situation can be somewhat complex, however. Depending on their origin, T cells may possess both pro-inflammatory and regulatory activity. Although this is somewhat confusing for immunologists trying to neatly organize cell types, it is clearly an advantage for the system to have sufficient plasticity that T cells can modulate their function as the situation develops.

One further mechanism of tolerance to be considered comes from the emergence of the *danger theory* of Polly Matzinger, or the infectious non-self model of Charles Janeway. Both of these theories considered that the important issue about whether an immune response was made against an antigen was not whether it was self or non-self, but *how* it was presented to the immune system. Antigens which are presented in the context of inflammation or infection (i.e. in a dangerous situation) will induce a response—but the same antigen presented in the absence of such signals will not. Immunologists have intuitively understood this for decades as they have made use of *adjuvants* (often bacterial products) in order to induce effective responses to vaccines. This now makes molecular sense as we understand much more about how such danger signals or PAMPs are sensed by the immune system and their impact on the antigen-presenting cell, as discussed in Chapter 2. It also makes sense given we now understand that the process of self-tolerance in the thymus is imperfect so many other layers of protection must be afforded.

One interesting, but fortunately rare, cause of auto-immunity is dysfunction of innate immunity in the disease Aicardi–Goutières Syndrome. Here there is failure to break down DNA effectively—so when cells die naturally their DNA is not disposed of appropriately. Free DNA within a cell is recognized as a danger signal through the pattern recognition receptor CGAS (see Chapter 2) and so this genetic defect leads to an enormous level of innate response—as if there were an ongoing virus infection. The ongoing inflammation induces auto-immunity, tissue damage, and severe disability in those affected.

The take-home message is that in the absence of innate signalling resulting from a pathogen or inflammation, an antigen should be ignored, whether it be self or non-self. This is an important scenario, as a self-reactive T cell sitting, for example, in a lymph node could very well receive signals through its TCR if its antigen is carried to it on a dendritic cell from a local tissue. If the dendritic cell has not received any signals regarding infection or inflammation, then the signal is safe, and the consequence is a phenomenon described as *anergy*—that is, loss of reactivity to further stimulation. Anergy leads to a failure to respond to future signals, and results from receiving only a TCR signal without accompanying co-stimulation or cytokines. It is a further, effective way to very specifically control auto-reactive cells in the periphery. Providing only partial signals to T cells is also a trick played by pathogens. HBV and HCV, for example, are viruses which induce an extremely poor innate response—thus although there is plenty

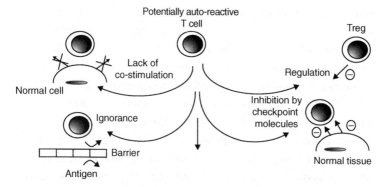

19. A number of different and overlapping mechanisms may lead to suppression of function or physical elimination of potentially auto-reactive T cells which have emerged from the thymus (i.e. peripheral tolerance).

of antigen presented to the immune system, responses cannot be properly initiated and it may take months to induce an effective T cell response. The mechanisms involved in peripheral tolerance are summarized in Figure 19.

Tolerance in specific organs: the liver and the placenta

The viruses HBV and HCV, mentioned earlier, also have a distinctive feature of targeting the liver, and it is no coincidence that they are able to set up long-term infections in this organ, as its immunologic profile is quite distinct from other tissues. The most striking data on this come from the work of Roy Calne in the 1960s, who developed a programme of liver transplantation in Cambridge. His work, described in the *Lancet* editorial 'Strange English Pigs', showed how transplantation without rejection was possible across conventional transplantation barriers. To understand the significance of this, it is first necessary to understand an important issue in transplantation of organs.

For other organs (e.g. kidney, heart, pancreas, and lung) there must be accurate matching between the recipient's MHC molecules and the donor's, otherwise there is a vigorous immune response. Although at first sight this may appear unexpected as the host's T cells are trained to recognize their own MHC molecules, it turns out that a foreign MHC presenting even an innocuous peptide will be bound and recognized as if it were a virus. In other words the overall shape of the foreign MHC is sufficient to engage T cell receptors and trigger an immune response. This response is further increased since graft will be put in through surgery, causing tissue damage and alerting the immune system through innate inflammatory responses. Thus in the normal case, if MHC matching between the donor and recipient does not occur, many T cells can be mobilized that home in on the graft, which causes major tissue damage and the graft to be rapidly rejected.

In the liver, however, MHC matching is not required. Furthermore, the recipients who have successfully engrafted a liver can also receive other organs from the same donor. In other words the liver graft has made them specifically tolerant to certain foreign antigens—the graft does not make them generally tolerant, only to the MHC molecules in the donor. In human liver transplants the same occurs—matching of donor recipient is only required in terms of blood type, and eventually the acceptance is so complete that in some cases no immune suppressive drugs are needed.

It is not clear exactly how the liver achieves this feat, but one mechanism is to present antigens with very limited co-stimulation. T cells which detect antigens under such circumstances fail to proliferate effectively and will undergo premature death. The liver contains its own specialist set of antigen-presenting cells in the form of liver sinusoidal endothelial cells which can avidly take up and present antigen. In the absence of inflammation these can effectively tolerize immune responses. Since the liver's blood supply is vast, and the cells move very slowly within the organ, these interactions are quite frequent and efficient.

One other interesting feature of the liver is that the endothelium is *fenestrated* (i.e. it has gaps or windows that allow the lymphocytes within the blood to contact the tissue cells—normally they would have to traverse the endothelium in order to do this). This feature means that naive T cells which do not possess the homing receptors that would allow them to enter tissue can potentially detect antigens presented in this organ. Efficient priming of the immune response normally occurs in the lymphoid organs, where it is supported by the correct blend of dendritic cells, co-stimulatory molecules, cytokines, and stromal support. The encounter of antigens for the first time in a peripheral tissue is likely to lead to partial and therefore ineffective activation as described earlier.

Why would the liver be designed this way? One argument is that we need to be tolerant to our own microbes living in the gut and the antigens from the food we eat. Since all the blood supply from the gut drains through the liver, presenting antigens in this *tolerizing* environment is one way to limit responses. Clearly this needs to be finely balanced since if a significant invasive pathogen comes via this route it is an ideal place to stop its spread before it reaches the rest of the body, and indeed the liver possesses an array of antimicrobial defences which are necessary to limit such spread—particularly an effective set of tissue-resident macrophages (Kupffer cells) which can engulf microbes. However, overall it appears the system is quite heavily regulated or dampened—the hepatitis viruses mentioned earlier clearly exploit this tolerant environment in order to establish viral persistence.

A further environment where it is essential to damp down immune responses which will naturally occur is in the setting of pregnancy. The foetus and placenta contain antigens which belong to both the mother and the father—unless the two are very closely related it really represents a mismatched graft and should be rejected. Clearly there is a set of tolerance mechanisms in place to prevent this occurring, including those described earlier. The entire immune system of the pregnant mother is in fact influenced by this process such that she is moderately immune-suppressed, and therefore at higher risk from certain infections such as varicella zoster (chickenpox) and malaria.

One interesting factor which can restrict immune responses in the placenta is modulation of immune metabolism. T cells require plentiful supplies of amino acids in order to function and one of these—tryptophan—can be seen to play an essential role, since specific loss of this molecule from their environment can turn off T cell activation. Restriction of tryptophan in the local environment is therefore a powerful way of arresting responses in the placenta, and this is done through up-regulation of an enzyme called indoleamine deoxygenase (IDO), which breaks it down effectively. IDO is not restricted to the placenta and indeed is activated in dendritic cells which allows them to regulate responses following activation. However, it has been shown that blocking IDO leads to immunological rejection of the foetus in mice, thus indicating it has an important role in foetal tolerance.

The liver has its own version of IDO (TDO) which is continuously generated and may serve to promote tolerance in that organ. Tryptophan is not the only amino acid manipulated in this way to modulate inflammation. Arginine is also essential and can be sequestered away from T cells to limit their function through the action of arginase, as found in tumours and in a specific group of regulatory cells related to macrophages described as myeloid suppressor cells.

Auto-immunity and inflammation

Having established the mechanisms which hold auto-immunity at bay, and having been introduced to some of the severe syndromes which occur if these fail, let us consider some common and complex auto-immune and inflammatory diseases. One of the best known of these is rheumatoid arthritis (RA), which leads to inflammation of the joints and ultimately their destruction, in severe cases, as well as being associated with inflammatory tissue damage to other organs. The cause of RA is not known, but let us consider one interesting hypothesis which pulls together many known strands.

The risk of RA is highly dependent on specific MHC molecules, particularly Class II molecules (such as HLA DRB1* 04). This indicates that presentation of specific peptides from these molecules is part of the cause of the disease. The disease is also clearly associated with the development of antibodies to a specific class of protein—*citrullinated* proteins. Citrulline is a modification of arginine which can occur during inflammation, for example, and by changing the shape of the antigenic protein it creates a new target for the immune system. Antibodies to citrullinated peptides are used as part of the diagnostic tests for RA. It is also seen very early, again suggesting it is linked to the cause of the disease. Smoking is also increasingly linked to RA—the risk of RA rises with both the duration and the intensity of smoking.

One idea therefore put forward by Lars Klareskog and colleagues is that smoking leads to the generation of citrullinated proteins which potentially form new targets for the immune response. In the presence of a *risk* HLA molecule, these new peptides are presented and tolerance is broken, followed by the development of antibodies to these modified targets. These auto-immune reactions can impact on both the lungs (which may show changes in RA, even if it is not clinically apparent) as well as the joints. It may be that a second hit is required to initiate the joint inflammation, since the antibodies can appear many years before the joint disease develops. Overall, this is an interesting idea which links the genetic and environmental factors driving RA, and also suggests that there are different variants of RA with different causes, since some individuals do not develop antibodies to citrullinated proteins. The factors involved in RA are summarized in Figure 20.

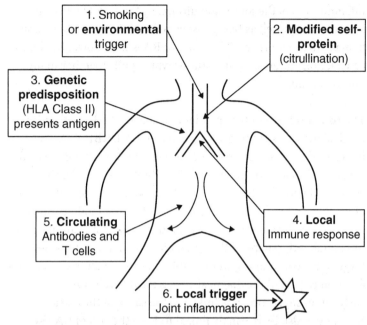

20. **A model for rheumatoid arthritis (RA) proposed incorporates some of the known genetic and environmental triggers. The inflammation can also be linked to development of disease symptoms outside the joints (e.g. in the lung or skin).**

Multiple sclerosis (MS) is a potentially devastating disease resulting from auto-immune responses occurring within the central nervous system. This inflammation leads to loss of the myelin sheath around nerves and thus loss of their function. It is typically an intermittent disease, with attacks, followed by a period of quiescence, but it can lead to cumulative disability over time. Like RA, it is also strongly linked to HLA Class II genes, in this case the DR2 complex (e.g. DRB1*1501), suggesting a role for T helper cells in its initiation. MS also has a very interesting connection between genetic and environmental causes. It is much more common in temperate climatic zones, such as northern Europe and the US (or early migration to those zones), much more common in women, and also increasingly linked to infection with EBV.

EBV is a very common infection throughout the globe, nearly ubiquitous in some settings, and MS is thought to occur in 2.5 million individuals, so it cannot be a simple relationship between cause and effect. One idea is that there is epitope mimicry between a peptide from EBV and one from the brain tissue (e.g. myelin basic protein)—this mimicry would only be seen when the peptide was presented by the risk MHC protein, explaining the genetic risk. Alternatively, EBV infection in the brain of a susceptible individual could reveal self-proteins to the immune response and break tolerance to self, by providing the necessary danger signals (as discussed earlier).

The latter idea may be extended by considering one explanation for the geography of this disease which relates to sunlight exposure. Lack of sunlight in regions away from the equator is linked to lower Vitamin D levels—this vitamin has an important regulatory role in the immune system, and low levels are associated with auto-immunity. Interestingly, genetic variants which affect the levels of Vitamin D made in the body have an impact on MS risk, strengthening this causative association. There are some complex interactions between sex hormones and the immune system, but lower testosterone levels may also influence overall immune reactivity and are also linked to enhanced MS disease progression.

Overall, a picture is emerging of a series of steps between initiation of inflammation in the brain and development of clinical disease—normally these can be well regulated through all the checkpoints described earlier, but a series of environmental and genetic risks can tip the balance in favour of disease if they accumulate unfavourably. Fortunately, by picking apart some of these genetic risks, the door is opened to potential new therapies (such as modulation of Vitamin D or sex hormone levels), in addition to the biologic agents that target the immune cell populations responsible, discussed in Chapter 7.

Another auto-immune disease with complex causes resulting from a gene–environment interaction is inflammatory bowel disease (IBD). IBD is in fact at least two diseases—Crohn's disease is associated with deep fissures in the bowel and can occur anywhere along the gastrointestinal tract (including, for example, the mouth as well as the small bowel), while ulcerative colitis can lead to very severe inflammation affecting the large bowel only. Both may in fact be associated with some inflammatory features outside the gut (in joints and skin, for example), and they share genetic risk factors with each other and with other auto-immune diseases of those organs (ankylosing spondylitis and psoriasis, respectively). This points to a common pathway for inflammation and possibly an overlapping causation.

While RA and MS affect organs where there is normally no microbial presence (sterile sites), IBD affects the gut, which is the home to trillions of bacteria as part of our normal gut flora or *microbiome*. A number of rare inherited genetic defects can lead to IBD. IL-10 is a cytokine which can powerfully suppress immune responses. Loss of this molecule or loss of its receptor and downstream signals leads to very early onset of the disease. These point to an important role for immune regulation in control of responses to the microbiome, and the prevailing model for IBD is that this fine balancing act breaks down, leading to continuing inflammation. The normal microbial content of the gut must be largely ignored by the immune system, even though if the same microbes moved only a few millimetres across the gut wall into the bloodstream they would represent a major health threat. There is likely a continuous process whereby any misplaced microbe is dealt with very efficiently without the need to activate a full inflammatory response—these aggressive responses are, however, readily brought into play if a real pathogen attempts invasion.

The genetics of IBD are very striking and point to two important strands leading to disease. First is the Type 17 defence axis which we encountered earlier in the context of surface defence against yeasts, and this is regulated by cytokines such as Interleukin 23 (IL-23). Variants in genes influencing this axis are linked to increased risk of IBD. Second, the innate immune response is also important, since a specific gene, NOD2, is involved and this is a pattern recognition receptor for bacteria. Failure to recognize and rapidly deal with relatively harmless *commensal* bacteria may promote ongoing immune responses in the gut and set up a vicious circle whereby gut damage leads to further exposure to bacteria in the host tissue (see Figure 21).

There are a number of interesting new approaches to suppressing such inflammation, for example specific blockade of cytokines and chemokines (discussed in Chapter 7 in more detail). The cause of the disease, however, is a poorly balanced relationship with one's own gut flora, and this has a much wider implication for human health.

Microbiome populations are very complex and only with new molecular techniques is it becoming possible to dissect out the

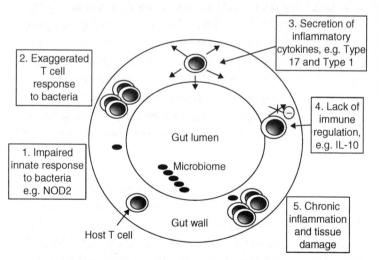

2. Exaggerated T cell response to bacteria

3. Secretion of inflammatory cytokines, e.g. Type 17 and Type 1

4. Lack of immune regulation, e.g. IL-10

1. Impaired innate response to bacteria e.g. NOD2

Gut lumen

Microbiome

5. Chronic inflammation and tissue damage

Host T cell

Gut wall

21. **Inflammatory bowel disease (IBD), Crohn's disease, and ulcerative colitis have a very strong genetic predisposition but also require an environmental trigger (likely the microbiome of the gut).**

vast array of species living within a single individual's gut. Many of these are not possible to culture with standard methods and have been ignored to date by microbiologists who naturally have focused on organisms that have been linked with disease. The relationship between host and microbiome has evolved over time as the flora are acquired after birth, and each individual will develop a slightly different balance. The flora also modulate the development of the immune response through exposure not only to PAMPs and bacterial antigens, but also to bacterial metabolic products, and this can have an important influence on the host immune response not only at the gut interface but also throughout the body.

This area of study has attracted a lot of attention recently, and different microbiome populations have been associated with different types of disease, from IBD, through RA and MS, to obesity, Parkinson's Disease, and Alzheimer's Disease. This type of research is still at a relatively early stage, so closely tying a specific change in a microbial population to a mechanism leading to a disease has been rarely achieved. However, if causality is proven, taking steps to modulate the gut microbiome may provide an interesting additional intervention to prevent or even treat a range of disorders. It should also be noted that the gut is not the only part of the body with its own microbiome—even within the gut this varies, but there are also bacterial commensals living in different regions of the skin and throat. These likely not only influence the local immune systems but have a potentially wider impact.

These three examples all show how different genetic and environmental triggers combine to increase the risk of auto-immune disease. Each individual risk may be relatively small, but the combination of risks serves to break down the security defences which have been set up through evolution to protect against auto-reactivity. One way of looking at this is that there are usually multiple layers of defence, and thus a number of things need to go wrong for auto-reactivity to cause problems. Given that the risks from each impact, genetic or environmental, tend to be rather small on their own, very large studies—usually of thousands of affected patients—are required to detect their effects. Fortunately, the genetic technologies and analysis of *big data* (huge stores of electronic health data) have reached a point where this is possible.

Allergy

Allergy is related to auto-immunity in the sense that it is a failure of the immune response to respond to normal cues, leading to an exaggerated and harmful response to inappropriate antigens. In this case the substance is not self, but it is harmless (non-dangerous) non-self. Through the mechanisms of tolerance described earlier, exposure to such an antigen, such as pollen, proteins from house dust mites, or food, should evoke minimal responsiveness. However, aberrant responses or hypersensitivity to such antigens is remarkably common and can be very dangerous.

The hallmark of allergy is the induction of a Type 2 immune response, driven by a specific set of T cells called Type 2 T cells (see Figure 22). Type 2 T cells tend to secrete lower levels of antiviral cytokines such as interferon-gamma and more of a distinct set of Interleukins (notably IL4, IL-5, and IL-13), which are able to stimulate quite different cell types and functions. Clearly these did not evolve simply to promote allergy—the driving force appears to be host defence against worms. Worm infection is more complex than bacterial, fungal, or viral, since the invading pathogen is multi-cellular and is orders of magnitude larger in size than the immune cells fighting it, and thus is not readily phagocytosed. Although in modern Western societies, encounters with worm infections are rare, in earlier stages of human evolution, worm infection would have represented an enormous burden—and it remains so in some parts of the world. Thus, a robust defence against worms is essential and requires a combination of effectors mobilized through the Type 2 response.

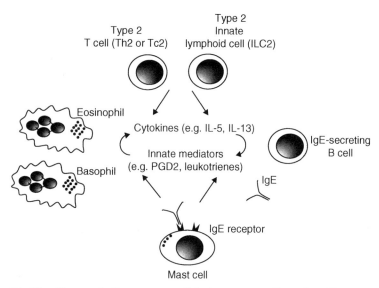

22. The diagram indicates some of the important cells and mediators involved in Type 2 responses. The triggering antigens which are recognized by Type 2 T cells and specific IgE include harmless proteins (e.g. from house dust mites) as well as drugs and insect venoms.

One key set of cells which are induced as part of this process are *eosinophils*. These are bone marrow derived and related to neutrophils, but possess a different content of granules and thus are readily distinguished. These granules contain specific, highly potent molecules which can digest and attack tissues, including worms—these include reactive oxygen species, protease enzymes, and pore-forming proteins that attack cell membranes. They also secrete a large set of mediators which recruit further cells to the site and activate them. Excess levels of eosinophils in the blood is one hallmark of worm infection—it is also a hallmark of allergy.

Another important mediator of allergy driven by the Type 2 response is the development of a particular type of antibody called the E class—*IgE*. Like high levels of eosinophils, high levels of IgE are associated strongly with allergy. IgE is no different from any other antibody at the antigen recognition end. However, the molecule is distinct in that it can activate a set of receptors present on specific subsets of immune cells called *mast cells*. If a mast cell with activated receptors encounters an antigen—for example, in the skin or airways—there is a rapid activation of the cell itself, resulting in a burst of inflammatory signals. Mast cell activation is highly potent as the cell contains pre-formed molecules, such as histamines, which leads to immediate inflammatory responses in the tissue—this is manifest as local swelling and irritation. Massive mast cell release can lead to very profound general effects—so-called *anaphylaxis*, where there may be a sudden drop in blood pressure, generalized swelling particularly of sensitive areas such as the face and tongue, and a rash. This response can be brought on by exposure to any antigen to which IgE has developed at sufficient levels, including proteins in insect stings, drugs, and food.

Allergic responses are commonly seen as organ-specific diseases, such as hay fever, asthma, or eczema. Often these are linked together within an individual or within families, and indeed there is a strong genetic predisposition to such diseases. Although many of the genes involved relate to the immune response, not all of them do. For eczema, mutations in the filaggrin gene lead to a subtle disruption of the skin barrier—exactly how this leads to allergy is not known, but it is likely that it allows exposure to more antigens or a change in the context in which the immune system encounters an antigen, thus raising its awareness and promoting a Type 2 response.

Other mutations affect molecules involved specifically in the activation of different cell subsets involved in the Type 2 reaction, for example CRTH2. CRTH2 is a surface receptor for prostaglandin D2—one of the important lipid mediators released by mast cells. CRTH2 is found on Type 2 T cells, on eosinophils, on basophils (which are closely related), and also on innate lymphoid cells which have a Type 2 bias. It is thus a distinct marker of the Type 2 subset and furthermore a target for drugs which can block prostaglandin signalling. Prostaglandins and their lipid relatives, leukotrienes, are involved in a range of inflammatory processes, and blockade of the action of leukotrienes by the drug Montelukast has long been used as a treatment for asthma.

Although a wide range of cells are involved in allergic responses, they share a few key pathways, and signalling molecules (such as Prostaglandin D2 or Interleukin 5), which are rather distinct from those encountered in other immune settings. This offers some hope that we can find treatments for asthma that are more targeted. Allergic asthma results from ongoing Type 2 responses in the lung, which lead to inflammation of the airways and constriction of the airways. These are related but distinct features. Currently treatment relies in most cases on the use of inhaled steroids to suppress local inflammation and compounds related to adrenaline to improve the airway constriction. However, if the disease is severe, steroids must be given at high doses orally or intravenously to keep the airways open, and this is associated with long-term side effects (bone thinning, immune suppression, weight gain).

Approaches to specifically turn off Type 2 responses which underpin this severe disease are still needed, although biologic agents which block, for example, Interleukin 5 represent one interesting approach. It is also possible in some cases of allergy to reprogramme the immune response and replace the Type 2 response with a less dangerous one. This can be done by a process of *desensitization* whereby a tiny dose of the antigen is given in the skin, and this dosing is repeated and built up over a long period of time. What is observed is that IgE levels (e.g. from bee venom) to the antigen drop, while IgG4 responses may replace these. IgG4 is an interesting molecule which has little activatory function and may serve as a blocking or inhibitory antibody. This therapy has in fact been in place for over a century, developed well before a clear understanding of the immune mechanisms was in place—but the same is true for vaccines.

There is still much to learn about allergy—for instance the reason why an individual develops a particular allergic response to a given antigen is not well understood. Like auto-immunity there will be a component from the genetic polymorphisms the person has inherited and the environment to which they are exposed, including their microbiome. One prevalent theory which suggests a specific role for environmental exposure is the *hygiene hypothesis*, whereby exposure to a high microbial burden in childhood reduces the chance of developing an allergy. This is somewhat controversial but has been put forward to explain the rise in allergic diseases in Western societies.

Certainly there are data which support the idea that the greater the diversity of pathogens to which children are exposed (e.g. living on a farm increases this substantially), the lower the risk of allergy. In a study of the Amish and Hutterite communities in the USA, it was found that although the two groups were very closely matched in many ways, the Amish children had a much lower incidence of asthma. It turns out that the Amish communities used traditional farming practices as opposed to the modern industrialized techniques adopted by the Hutterites, and the environment in Amish homes was characterized by a much greater range and burden of microbes. How exactly this microbial exposure may work, by diverting or training the immune response, is not fully understood, but it is another example of how the microbiome may have a pervasive influence on immune development.

Chapter 7

The immune system v2.0: biological and immune therapies

In the previous chapters we have discussed the basic building blocks of the immune system, how they work as a team, and what happens when the teamwork breaks down. This basic knowledge can be applied, however, to influence outcomes of disease—both immunological and beyond. In this chapter we will discuss three major inter-related areas where our knowledge of immunology is being applied to current challenges: boosting immunity in the case of vaccines, harnessing immunity for cancer treatment, and the development of novel treatments for blocking immunity and auto-immunity. We will also look at the issues linked to the ageing immune response and how these may be corrected to treat or prevent disease.

Boosting immunity and vaccines

First let's consider how to boost immune responses, and perhaps the most obvious application is in the field of vaccines. Vaccines have had an enormous impact on human health for centuries, and the immunological principles which underlie them are increasingly well understood—but we still lack effective vaccines for major infections such as HIV, TB, and malaria. Why is this and what can be done? What these three infections have in common, and is also common to other complex vaccine targets such as HCV and CMV, is their capacity to persist. Infections such as influenza,

Haemophilus influenzae, and measles tend not to set up a persistent infection in an otherwise healthy host and the immunity induced is robust—so a vaccine approach which generates high levels of antibody against the prevailing strains can provide *protective immunity.* For influenza the challenge is to establish which strains pose the threat, and there is a wide range with some avian strains being very dangerous indeed if they cross into human hosts, but the issue is nevertheless the same. For the current influenza vaccines, providing the proteins derived from the relevant virus type circulating that season (using virus grown on chicken eggs), together with an adjuvant, which enhances the innate immune response, is usually sufficient to induce protective levels of neutralizing antibody. For measles, which is an attenuated version of the natural virus, this immunity is lifelong.

However, as we have seen for HIV, generation of antibodies against the viral envelope can neutralize some strains but is readily escaped by others and provides only limited protection. One trial (RV144, in Thailand) which was designed to induce antibodies against the HIV envelope has shown partial success in preventing infection and has raised hopes that effective antibodies can be raised, but there is a long way to go before this can be used, as the level of protection was only 30 per cent. Further attempts to optimize the antigen used, and to focus the antibody response on regions which can neutralize multiple variants, may enhance this.

Alternative approaches are hoped to harness the T cell response in providing protection. This would be relying on the CD8+ T cells to clear infection from already infected cells and so is quite a different approach from that used in the vaccines mentioned earlier. Such approaches have been tried, but unsuccessfully, and there were concerns raised that the vaccines may even increase the chances of infection in people with HIV. It may be that the T cells need to be targeted to the right peptides in the virus.

One approach from the lab of Louis Picker has been to use CMV as a *vector* (carrier virus) to deliver the HIV proteins. The CMV used in these experiments can disable some aspects of MHC Class I presentation, which apparently forces the immune system to use alternative presenting molecules, in this case a molecule in humans known as HLA-E.

HLA-E is not polymorphic and presents a limited set of peptides, normally to NK cells—but in the context of this vaccine, which to date has only been used in monkeys, it can present viral peptides. The immune responses to these peptides are very strong and quite distinct from the normal immune response, and they can be remarkably effective in suppressing infection. These experiments provide some proof-of-principle that T cell-based approaches could work, if this can be translated safely into human studies.

Virally vectored vaccines—that is, vaccines where the target pathogen is presented to the immune system using another virus (see Figure 23)—do have huge potential. It is possible to engineer safe viruses which can present the target antigens (from e.g. TB, Zika virus, or Ebola) to the immune system, and some of these (e.g. adenoviruses) are able to prime extremely vigorous immune responses. This means it is not necessary to grow the pathogens in the lab, and the immune response can in theory be targeted specifically to the regions of interest. It is also possible to use DNA itself as a vaccine—the injected DNA will be used by the cell to generate the protein of interest and there may be a sufficient innate response to the vaccine to prime new T and B cells. DNA vaccines work very effectively in mice but relatively poorly in humans—indeed one of the handicaps of this area is that many vaccine approaches that work well in the laboratory fail to induce strong immune responses in human volunteers.

So, some of the difficulties in generating vaccines against complex pathogens arise from failure to understand what type of immunity is protective and what target to hit, and some arise from failing to

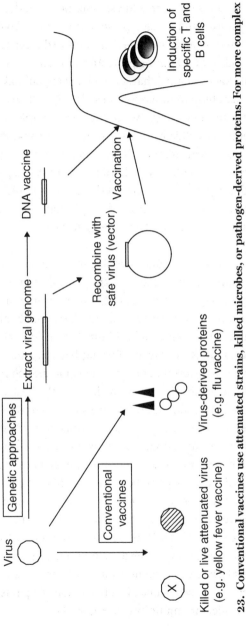

23. Conventional vaccines use attenuated strains, killed microbes, or pathogen-derived proteins. For more complex or dangerous pathogens a genetic approach may provide an alternative vaccine strategy.

be able to induce immune responses using current approaches. Of the two, the latter is easier to address since better understanding of innate responses and antigen presentation coupled with an increasingly diverse array of molecular tools to deliver antigens could solve this issue. Defining protective immunity and trying to reproduce it exactly is much harder—even using animal models which represent human disease—and so it may still be a matter of trial and error in some cases. Two particularly complex diseases which currently lack effective vaccine strategies are malaria and TB. These share some features with HIV: malaria has very high levels of variability, which make it very hard for the host's responses to keep up with the pathogen, while TB sets up a reservoir of latent infection antigens which is very hard to eliminate and represents a continuous threat of potential reinfection.

Immunity to malaria is actually possible to develop through continuous exposure over time—infection of children and infants is very dangerous and associated with severe illness, but adults from communities in areas where malaria is endemic, such as in sub-Saharan Africa, may suffer minimal or no clinical impact from a malarial infection. Much effort has been expended in defining the mechanisms that limit the infection in such individuals (interestingly such effective immunity is lost if the individuals move away from an endemic area) and a vaccine—RTS,S—has been generated as a result. This vaccine, which uses HBV to present malarial antigens to the immune system is, however, only partially effective in infants and the effect wears off over time, so there is certainly more work to be done here. Malaria parasites have a complex lifestyle which includes a key stage passing through the liver after the mosquito bite, before emerging and passing into red blood cells. Where the infection in the liver can be blocked this provides very effective immunity. Approaches to direct anti-malaria T cell responses into the liver using virally vectored vaccines or even whole, irradiated malaria parasites can provide quite efficient immunity (see Figure 24).

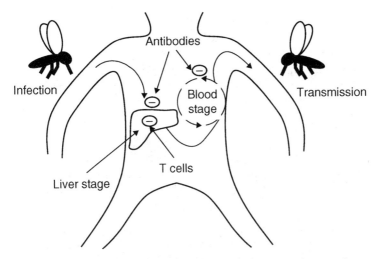

Infection

Liver stage

Antibodies

Blood
stage

T cells

Transmission

24. Malaria parasites are transmitted from biting mosquitoes and must enter the liver in order to establish infection. Antibodies and T cells induced by vaccines and natural exposure can block this process at different points.

TB is caused by Mtb (see Chapter 2) and spread largely by aerosol droplets from infected individuals presenting with a productive cough. The organism is present in about a third of the world's population, and the key step in its life cycle is its ability to set up long-term latency in macrophages, the major cell it infects. The bacterium is able to manipulate the intracellular environment of the macrophage to enhance its survival and evade immune elimination. Since it is intracellular, the key immune responses are delivered by T cells, and deficits in T cell immunity can lead to reactivation of TB. T cells secrete cytokines such as interferon-gamma and TNF-alpha which activate the macrophages and enhance the elimination. This cross-talk between T cells and macrophages leads to the development of a *granuloma*—a complex mass of immune cells at the centre of which is embedded the bacterium driving the response (see Figure 25).

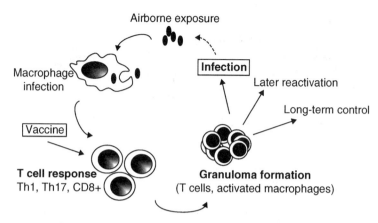

Airborne exposure

Macrophage infection

Infection

Later reactivation

Long-term control

Vaccine

T cell response
Th1, Th17, CD8+

Granuloma formation
(T cells, activated macrophages)

25. *Mycobacterium tuberculosis* (Mtb) is taken up by macrophages. In most cases Mtb persists in a granuloma and it can reactivate at a later date. If T cell immunity is poor, further spread of Mtb within the lung can occur.

A T cell vaccine against TB has existed for nearly a century in the form of BCG developed at the Pasteur Institute in Paris. This vaccine—which is based on an attenuated strain of TB developed in culture—does indeed generate high levels of T cell response against Mtb antigens. It has also been shown to be highly effective in preventing disease in infants, where it can be very severe, spreading throughout the body including to the brain (i.e. meningitis). However, BCG is much less obviously effective in adults and no new vaccine has been developed since. The reasons for this are not yet clear, but one issue is that we do not yet know what the key mediators of protection are and therefore what the vaccine should target. Once we have a clear target the methods to induce T cell immunity in humans are now well advanced and so new TB vaccine strategies could provide a breakthrough prevention of this major, global health problem.

It is clearly important to develop new vaccines. One high priority is RSV (see also Chapter 4) which is a widespread, indeed ubiquitous, virus to which we are all exposed and which causes severe disease in young infants. A vaccine against RSV would be of enormous benefit around the world, but an attempt to make one in the 1960s was associated with increased disease and also death in those vaccinated. It is likely that this resulted from an aberrant Type 2 immune response generated against the vaccine, which was developed from a live virus that had been rendered inactive by a chemical, formalin. Thus an enhanced immune response was not protective but rather led to hypersensitivity to the virus and increased lung inflammation.

Further attempts to make vaccines against RSV are nevertheless underway, using our increased knowledge of the immune system to avoid this dangerous problem either by using viral vectors to deliver the RSV antigens, or by vaccinating the mother, allowing her to pass on her boosted IgG antibodies to the infant and thus passively protect them. The infant's levels of protective antibody will drop over time but this means infection at the most vulnerable age can be avoided. There is emerging evidence that RSV also causes disease in the elderly, when immune responses wane (discussed later in this chapter), and here vaccines to boost antibodies and T cells against RSV could prevent serious infection in this age group.

Overall the development of vaccines against common diseases has saved countless lives and will continue to do so—they not only protect the individual vaccinated but beyond that provide *herd immunity*, limiting the spread of serious infections. This issue of herd immunity has come to the fore in recent controversies over the use of specific vaccines. Because vaccines are given to healthy individuals, the benefits of protection have to be weighed against the risks of possible adverse effects. Fortunately, because the impact of some of these infections is very great, and the risk from the vaccines is small, this equation comes down well in favour of benefit. If the same balance and outcome can be achieved using the next generation of vaccines against major pathogens such as those mentioned in this chapter, this has the potential to impact positively on millions of lives.

Harnessing immunity and cancer immunotherapy

Boosting immunity is not only of relevance to infections but also to cancer (Figure 26). One of the most exciting breakthroughs in the last decade has been the development of new techniques to harness anti-cancer immune responses for patient benefit. The evidence from HIV (and other immunosuppressive states) already suggested that the immune response plays a major role in controlling cancers, primarily those that are driven by viruses. However, most cancers do not contain viral proteins as potential targets but are simply mutated versions of self. Given the layers of tolerance described in the last chapter, immune responses to self are highly attenuated—additionally cancers behave somewhat like infections, undergoing selection to avoid elimination.

Thus developing an effective cellular immune response against cancers could be considered a very difficult proposition. On the

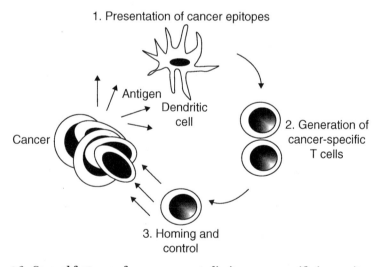

26. **Several features of cancers serve to limit cancer-specific immunity. These negative effects work both on the induction of the immune response (dendritic cell) and also at the effector stage (in the tumour micro-environment).**

other hand there have been intermittent successes in this field, where some patients have demonstrated a striking response to vaccination or the transfer of specific T cells, which has led to continued optimism regarding this approach. In looking at outcomes from cancer, and studying the cells and genes in the tumours themselves, there are signs that the greater the immune response in the tumour, the better the survival of the patient. Recent data used to examine outcomes from thousands of patients with thirty different types of cancer revealed that the single gene in the tumours most closely linked to a good outcome was an immune gene—KLRB1—encoding for CD161, a molecule expressed on subsets of T cells and NK cells with enhanced functions.

What might such T cells be recognizing within a cancer? One answer lies in analysing the cancer itself, which is a result of genetic mutations in the DNA of the host cells. Each time a significant mutation is made, a new peptide target is created that was not present in the thymus and where tolerance has not been previously induced. If such a peptide can be bound to the patient's MHC molecule and presented to the T cell, then it can represent a *neo-epitope*—a suitable target for recognition and killing of the tumour cell. Interestingly, some tumours where this process of mutation is accelerated (due to loss of proofreading of the cell's replication machinery) are actually better controlled, and associated with a more vigorous immune response—likely targeting the large set of neo-epitopes generated. With new methods of sequencing of cancer genomes now available, it is possible to identify the neo-epitopes which are present in an individual patient's cancer. In principle targeting these with a vaccine approach could lead to bespoke cancer therapies.

However, the T cell responses also need to overcome the tolerance effects present in tissues and in particular the checkpoints provided by inhibitory molecules. This is the area where the recent ability to block such checkpoints with monoclonal antibodies has had the biggest impact. Blockade of inhibitory molecules such as PD1 and CTLA4 can have a huge impact on cancer control—in combination (and without other treatment) these can lead to marked extension of disease-free survival in patients with advanced melanoma, one of the most aggressive forms of cancer. Melanomas are an interesting tumour as they possess well-established targets for the immune system and have been known to respond to immune therapies in the past. Checkpoint blockade is now being applied to a range of other tumour types, such as lung cancer and renal cancers. The downside, as may be expected, is the induction of auto-immune phenomena (gut inflammation is particularly common), but given the prognosis from the cancer itself, these can be largely accepted if appropriately controlled.

There are a number of mechanisms which regulate T cell functions in healthy tissues and tumours, so it is hoped that this success can be built upon to provide a range of options to liberate anti-tumour responses in future—but this approach does depend on the presence of a potentially active T cell response. Thus it may also be coupled with efforts to boost the anti-tumour response through vaccines (as described in this chapter) or using infusions of lymphocytes—so-called cellular therapies.

One novel approach to cellular therapy is the creation of so-called chimeric antigen receptor (CAR-T) cells, where the TCR has been engineered to respond specifically to the patient's cancer. This can target new T cells to the cancer where they are activated and display effector functions. This targeting can be made exquisitely specific by engineering an antibody domain onto the TCR—thus this does not rely on peptide presentation of a processed peptide, but rather expression of a cancer antigen on the cell surface. Antibody binding to such targets is very specific and very strong. This approach is also interesting as the T cells may remain circulating and provide long-term protection against recurrence. Similar approaches are being attempted using engineered soluble

TCRs which have been selected for their ability to very strongly bind to a tumour target (normally TCRs are relatively weak, since strong binders are eliminated in the thymus). These can be designed so that when engaged with their target they can recruit effector T cells and activate them directly at the site of the tumour, thus hugely increasing the numbers of cells involved in the anti-tumour response.

Blocking immunity and biological therapies

On the one hand, our understanding of the mechanisms of tolerance can allow us to break them and enhance inflammation in the case of cancer responses. On the other, our knowledge of the basic mechanisms of inflammation can suggest strategies to block auto-immune responses. The most interesting new approach to such a blockade relies on adapting the immune response itself to generate *biological therapies* based on monoclonal antibodies, developed by César Milstein and Georges Köhler, who shared the Nobel Prize for this work with Niels Jerne.

Monoclonal antibodies are derived from the normal antibody response, which contains many different forms of antibody response even to the same antigen. To make a single, purified form, Köhler and Milstein fused B cells with *immortalized* cancer cells (i.e. cells which can keep on dividing and therefore growing indefinitely in the lab) to create a series of *hybridomas*. These immortalized cells all secrete an antibody, but each cell makes an antibody of a distinct and unique design. By doing this at scale, and then screening the resultant hybridomas for binding to the antigen of choice (in the original study it was sheep red blood cells, but it can be anything which evokes an antibody response), it is possible to select those hybridomas with the correct specificity. Since hybridomas are immortalized this allows immunologists to make almost unlimited quantities of highly purified and specific antibodies to targets of their choice. This technology is still used, although newer, more flexible alternatives have been developed.

Monoclonal antibodies allow for precise blockading of specific aspects of the immune system or targeting of pathogens. Although these tools were developed by Milstein and Köhler in the 1970s, it took some time for their therapeutic potential to be realized. The leader of this pack was the development of monoclonal antibodies to Tumor Necrosis Factor alpha (TNFa). This molecule is highly pro-inflammatory and is involved in many and diverse auto-immune and inflammatory responses as well as being critical in host defence. Monoclonal therapy for TNFa was tested initially in the context of sepsis—a severe condition of bloodstream infections associated with a very high mortality rate. Like many therapies for this condition, it was not successful. However, Marc Feldman and Ravinder Maini, who had been working on TNFa in RA and had shown the effects of blockade in the test tube, were able to repurpose this treatment—known as *Infliximab*—in a small trial of patients with this disabling condition. The results from this trial in 1992 were remarkably effective, with a substantial proportion of patients benefiting from the monoclonal antibody, and paving the way for a flood of such biological treatments in the following decades. TNFa blockade (using Infliximab and other biological approaches) is now used in treating a wide range of inflammatory conditions, including IBD (Crohn's disease and ulcerative colitis), ankylosing spondylitis, and psoriatic arthritis.

Biological therapies allow the pinpoint blockade of specific pathways involved in inflammation, thus avoiding the use of very broad immunosuppressive therapies such as steroids. However, there are side effects which may be predicted from the role of these molecules in host defence. TNFa is critically important in the control of TB, and even though other immune defence mechanisms remain intact, those treated with this agent are at risk of reactivating this infection. Also, although the molecule has been engineered to be 'humanized' (it was originally developed in a mouse), it can still, in some patients, attract an antibody response which limits its effectiveness. Not all patients with RA (or the other diseases mentioned) respond to such drugs. This

The Immune System

suggests that although RA appears to be one disease, there may be different underlying mechanisms at work in different patients—so further stratification of patients for these expensive and potentially dangerous therapies is needed—a common theme in modern medicine.

Beyond TNFa, a number of other cytokine pathways can be targeted by monoclonal antibodies. The Type 17 pathway has been mentioned previously as a contributor to inflammatory disease, as well as protecting against infection by bacteria and yeasts. Blockade of IL-23, a cytokine that promotes such responses, is also effective in inflammatory diseases of the joints and bowel. Interestingly blockade of IL-17 itself is effective in treating ankylosing spondylitis, an inflammatory disease of the spine, and also in psoriasis—diseases which share a number of genetic risk factors with each other and with IBD. However, IL-17 blockade in IBD actually made the inflammation worse, possibly by reducing the host response to bacteria and thus accentuating the original injury. In some ways, therefore, these clinical studies are experiments themselves, revealing further aspects of the underlying disease once one pathway has been blocked; or revealing the role of a specific pathway in host defence.

The ability to target and specifically block an inflammatory pathway in patients with chronic inflammation has been hugely attractive to scientists and companies, and the list of products now in trial or available for use is very long. Monoclonal antibodies to block other inflammatory cytokines or their receptors such as for Interleukins 1b and 6 can also be used to treat arthritis and may represent alternatives for those who do not respond to TNFa blockade. Blockade of IL-5 and potentially IL-13 represent interventions for allergy and asthma. There is plenty of potential to influence these inflammatory conditions, although the development of such agents is very costly and so care must be taken in choosing the right targets.

Other approaches based on monoclonal therapy include cell depletion—indeed Campath 1, targeting T cells through their surface receptor CD52, was one of the first such treatments developed by Herman Waldmann in Cambridge. Now known as Alemtuzumab, this depleting antibody can have a substantial impact on the course of MS and is one of the few therapies which is really effective in this disease. Depletion of cells using monoclonals can also be effective in cancer. Alemtuzumab can be used for specific lymphatic tumours, to destroy the proliferating lymphocytes, but more importantly targeting of the CD20 molecule by the antibody Rituximab on B cells is a powerful treatment for a range of lymphomas. Rituximab, by depleting B cells (most of which express the CD20 molecule and are targets for the drug), can also reset the immune system and can be used to turn off antibody responses in RA and a range of auto-immune conditions. The story for these molecules, like that of Infliximab mentioned earlier, is informative—although introduced for a single condition or application, they can be turned to a variety of uses, including in relatively rare or 'orphan' conditions where specific drugs are unlikely to be developed.

Monoclonal antibodies and biological therapies can also be used to block the migration of cells to specific tissues. Vedolizumab is a blocker of specific *integrins* used to allow cells to home in on the gut where it is active in the treatment of IBD. Natulizumab is a related molecule but it impacts on the homing action of lymphocytes to both gut and brain, and can be used to treat MS. Failure to allow lymphocytes to survey the brain tissue, however, does not come without risk, since rare cases of a severe viral infection caused by JC virus can occur. This is also seen in advanced HIV patients, linked to profound immunosuppression and with a very poor outcome. Such viral reactivations do occur in other settings, and while some are predictable and preventable (such as reactivation of chronic HBV), many are not, and care must be taken even with such targeted therapies (see Figure 27).

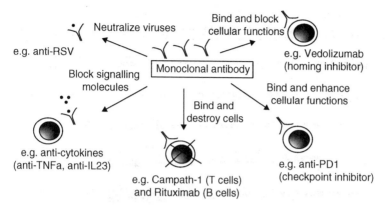

27. Monoclonal antibodies allow for precise blockade of specific aspects of the immune system or targeting of pathogens. The ability to bind and kill cells can be used for immunotherapy and cancer therapy.

Turning off immune responses is not only required for inflammatory diseases but also for transplantation, and here monoclonal antibodies also play a role. Additionally, attempts have been made to induce tolerance using a range of techniques. One interesting idea based on cell therapy is to transfer in regulatory T cells. CD4+ T cells which express high levels of the IL-2 receptor CD25, marking out Tregs, can be sorted from peripheral blood, cultured in the laboratory, and transfused into the recipient. These cells may also be treated in vitro to enhance their ability to suppress. In pre-clinical studies this approach has been highly effective and there is much enthusiasm to translate it into human use, even though there will be many practical barriers to overcome. Treg therapy may also have a role in auto-immune diseases and potentially has the advantage of providing a relatively specific attenuation of the aberrant immune response without the risk of severe infection.

Inflammation and ageing ('inflammageing')

Finally, looking to the future, one issue we currently face is that of diseases of ageing, and in these the immune response may need

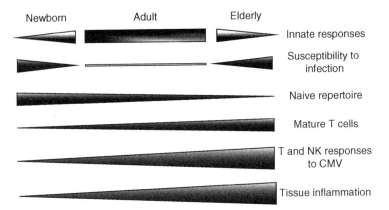

Newborn   Adult   Elderly

Innate responses

Susceptibility to infection

Naive repertoire

Mature T cells

T and NK responses to CMV

Tissue inflammation

28. Ageing is associated with many immunological changes which affect susceptibility to infection and regulation of inflammation. CMV infection drives very strong immune responses and has been associated with some of these effects.

tuning either up or down (see Figure 28). Alzheimer's disease is not considered an auto-immune disease like RA or MS, but there is increasing evidence, from studies of those affected and genetic analysis of large populations, that the immune response is involved. TREM2 is one such gene which is implicated in Alzheimer's disease and appears to influence the function of microglial cells—related to macrophages—in the brain. Exactly how TREM2 influences the development or progression of the dementia process is not currently understood, but it provides a potential new therapeutic opportunity to intervene in this devastating and prevalent illness.

Ageing itself may be accelerated by inflammation—so-called 'inflammageing'. This is a very complicated area because a number of factors are involved and distinguishing healthy ageing from premature senescence is not simple. One factor which may play a role is chronic inflammation due to infection. A culprit in many studies is CMV, a virus carried by most of the world's population and one where its capacity to lie dormant and then reactivate means that continuous immune surveillance is required. This in itself leads to a marked skewing of immune responses due to the number of lymphocytes recruited to this effort, and has been linked to premature senescence of the immune system, with loss of responsiveness. There is accruing data that loss of control over CMV, in a subset of individuals, leads to viral reactivation and inflammation. Since the virus is able to survive in the linings of blood vessels (endothelial cells), this could contribute to vascular disease. Further studies with large populations to address this specific hypothesis are needed—if this is indeed found to be true, then it may provide an interesting opportunity to interrupt the process of ageing.

Furthermore, developing vaccine strategies and other interventions to maintain an effective immune response in an ageing population will be of increasing importance in future. One recently explored idea is to focus on the metabolism of immune cells, specifically a process known as *autophagy*, or self-eating. Autophagy is a mechanism for recycling cell contents in order to maintain cell survival and is triggered by starvation. Much data have accrued to show that stimulating autophagy can improve lifespan. In the case of lymphocytes, autophagy is required to maintain long-lived memory—in one experiment, triggering autophagy in aged mice, which had markedly impaired T cell memory, using a molecule called spermidine, led to a marked improvement in memory T cell responses. This suggests that immune ageing processes are at least partially reversible and that simple interventions (spermidine, for example, is found in food) could assist this rejuvenation process. Autophagy can also be induced by many other means, including calorie restriction and exercise. So there may be multiple ways to influence this critical pathway and boost the ageing immune system. There are likely other pathways involved that limit immunity or immune regulation with age, but which are currently poorly explored.

Interestingly, autophagy is highly regulated by diet and exercise. The overall impact of nutritional status on such basic cellular processes is likely very important and the role of metabolic regulation of the immune system is of great significance. For example, micronutrients such as vitamins and minerals may modulate effector vs regulatory functions of T cells. Diabetes, which is an increasing problem in Western ageing populations, is linked with depression of immune function and increased susceptibility to infection. Further mechanistic and clinical studies are needed to better define whether specific interventions in diet and lifestyle can impact on immune responses and inflammatory processes in populations of all ages.

The future of the immune system

In this book we have examined the basic building blocks of the immune response, as we have inherited them through evolution, and how they coordinate their functions to balance aggression (against dangerous pathogens) with tolerance (of self and the microbiome). The job is normally done so well that we ignore its daily impact on our lives—only noticing it when it is impaired. In the first chapter, we discussed how the immune system involves the whole body and how we are increasingly aware that inflammatory processes are involved in many diseases, from heart disease through to cancer and dementia.

Evolution likely tuned our immune system to get us through only the first few decades of life so that the issues discussed earlier in this chapter may be a consequence of this early-age bias. The diseases we face globally still include many infectious challenges—such as HIV, malaria, and TB. Prevention and cure of these diseases will rely on better understanding of the targets of the immune system and on developing more practical systems for the induction of protective T and B cell immunity. This is an extension of the work that has been going on since Jenner and then Pasteur, the pioneers of vaccination, with increasing levels of refinement, driven by better understanding of basic immunology and microbiology. Here, harnessing the immune system through vaccine development has been enormously successful.

The diseases of the 21st century, particularly in the developed world, are dominated by cardiovascular disease and cancer, with dementia and diseases of old age emerging as population structures change. This is a different challenge for immunologists, but since the immune system involves the whole body and many important pathologies it is a challenge that must be met. The ability to specifically block inflammatory pathways—using small-molecule drugs or biological molecules based on monoclonal antibody technology—provides us with an important set of tools to modulate immune responses in these new settings. Given the enormous advances these approaches have made in classical auto-immune and inflammatory diseases such as RA and IBD, the new set of challenges can be approached with some optimism. Tuning or retraining the immune system to operate effectively in old age—that is, boosting immunity against infection while preventing chronic inflammation—is too complex a task for those in this field to tackle alone, and will need input from those in many other fields. However, as we dissect the immunological pathways involved in such diseases this will continue to provide new opportunities for treatment and ultimately prevention of these and other such conditions facing all of us as individuals and as a society.

Further reading

Books

Daniel M. Davis (2014) *The Compatibility Gene* (Penguin).

Arthur M. Silverstein (2009) *A History of Immunology*, 2nd edition (Academic Press).

Kenneth Murphy (2014) *Janeway's Immunobiology*, 8th edition (Garland Science).

Raif Geha and Luigi Notarangelo (2016) *Case Studies in Immunology—A Clinical Companion*, 7th edition (Garland Science).

Lauren Sompayrac (2012) *How the Immune System Works*, 4th edition (Blackwell Science).

Abul Abbas, Andrew H. Lichtman, and Shiv Pillai (2014) *Cellular and Molecular Immunology*, 8th edition (Saunders).

Peter Parham (2014) *The Immune System*, 4th edition (Garland Science).

Gordon MacPherson and Jon Austyn (2012) *Exploring Immunology—Concepts and Evidence*, 1st edition (Wiley VCH).

Warren E. Levinson (2014) *Review of Medical Microbiology and Immunology*, 13th edition (McGraw-Hill).

David Male, Jonathan Brostoff, David Roth, and Ivan Roitt (eds) (2012) *Immunology*, 8th edition (Saunders).

William Paul (2012) *Fundamental Immunology*, 7th edition (Lippincott Williams and Wilkins).

David Warrell, Tim Cox, and John Firth (eds) (2010) *Oxford Textbook of Medicine*, 5th edition (Oxford University Press). (Chapter 5, 'Immune Mechanisms', ed. Graham Ogg.)

Reviews

The field of immunology moves fast. The following journals publish up-to-date review articles on the subjects covered in this book, listed on PubMed (<https://www.ncbi.nlm.nih.gov/pubmed>):

Advances in Immunology <http://www.sciencedirect.com/science/bookseries/00652776>.
Annual Review of Immunology <http://www.annualreviews.org/journal/immunol>.
Current Opinion in Immunology <https://www.journals.elsevier.com/current-opinion-in-immunology>.
Immunological Reviews <http://onlinelibrary.wiley.com/journal/10.1111/(ISSN)1600-065X>.
Nature Reviews Immunology <http://www.nature.com/nri/index.html>.
Nature Reviews Microbiology <http://www.nature.com/nrmicro/index.html>.
Trends in Immunology <https://www.journals.elsevier.com/trends-in-immunology/>.

See also

R. M. Zinkernagel (1996) 'Immunology Taught by Viruses', *Science* 271: 173–8.

R. E. Phillips (2002) 'Immunology Taught by Darwin', *Nature Immunology* 3: 987–9.

M. M. Davis (2012) 'Immunology Taught by Humans', *Science Translational Medicine* 4: 117fs2. doi: 10.1126/scitranslmed. 3003385.

J. L. Casanova, L. Abel, and L. Quintana-Murci (2013) 'Immunology Taught by Human Genetics', *Cold Spring Harbor Symposia on Quantitative Biology* 78: 157–72. doi: 10.1101/sqb.2013.78.019968.

"牛津通识读本"已出书目

古典哲学的趣味	福柯	地球
人生的意义	缤纷的语言学	记忆
文学理论入门	达达和超现实主义	法律
大众经济学	佛学概论	中国文学
历史之源	维特根斯坦与哲学	托克维尔
设计，无处不在	科学哲学	休谟
生活中的心理学	印度哲学祛魅	分子
政治的历史与边界	克尔凯郭尔	法国大革命
哲学的思与惑	科学革命	民族主义
资本主义	广告	科幻作品
美国总统制	数学	罗素
海德格尔	叔本华	美国政党与选举
我们时代的伦理学	笛卡尔	美国最高法院
卡夫卡是谁	基督教神学	纪录片
考古学的过去与未来	犹太人与犹太教	大萧条与罗斯福新政
天文学简史	现代日本	领导力
社会学的意识	罗兰·巴特	无神论
康德	马基雅维里	罗马共和国
尼采	全球经济史	美国国会
亚里士多德的世界	进化	民主
西方艺术新论	性存在	英格兰文学
全球化面面观	量子理论	现代主义
简明逻辑学	牛顿新传	网络
法哲学：价值与事实	国际移民	自闭症
政治哲学与幸福根基	哈贝马斯	德里达
选择理论	医学伦理	浪漫主义
后殖民主义与世界格局	黑格尔	批判理论